Rheumatoid Hand Surgery

A Colour Atlas of
Rheumatoid Hand Surgery

Kenneth M. Backhouse
OBE, VRD, MRCS Eng., LRCP London
Reader in Applied Anatomy, Royal College
of Surgeons of England; Surgeon, Hand Unit,
Royal London Homeopathic Hospital

Stewart H. Harrison
FRCS Eng.; FRCS, LDS, RCS Edin.; Consultant
Plastic Surgeon, Mount Vernon Hospital, Northwood;
Past President, British Association of Plastic Surgeons;
Past President, British Society of Surgery of the Hand

Ralph T. Hutchings
Chief Medical Laboratory Scientific Officer,
Institute of Basic Medical Sciences,
Royal College of Surgeons of England

Wolfe Medical Publications Ltd

Contents

Preface

The medical authors of this book have each spent many years in the study and surgical treatment of the hand in rheumatoid disease and the allied arthroses. It is designed as an operative surgery book based on our joint experience. Alternative methods of surgery certainly exist, but have been omitted as they are not practised by ourselves; this does not necessarily mean they are less effective than those described. Even with two authors there are conflicts of opinion, but as Rainsford Mowlem once said; in plastic surgery there will always be six different ways of doing a particular operation and the best six surgeons in the world will all have similar results with different methods.

There is no doubt that this field of surgery is difficult and should not be undertaken lightly. This is not so much a matter of technical difficulty but of understanding and assessing the position of surgery in a generalized disease which should be treated with the rheumatologist.

Being an operative surgery book it is designed to be complementary to such excellent books as that by Adrian Flatt (*The care of the rheumatoid hand*, C.V. Mosby Company, St. Louis 1974) which deal more fully with the hand in relation to rheumatoid disease. Nevertheless it has been considered essential to include rather more general detail than is usual in operative surgery books, because of the nature of the conditions.

Secondly it is not enough to be good at hand surgery but familiar with normal anatomy and the altered anatomy resulting from the disease; the functions of the hand and the abnormalities of function. It is necessary to know what the normal hand can do and what each individual patient can or cannot do as a result of the disabling disease. Surgery then is one part of the work of a treatment team which includes the rheumatologist, occupational and physiotherapists as well as the surgeon and his operative and nursing colleagues.

It is hoped that our joint experiences will prove of some value to those who are already knowledgeable in the treatment of these conditions and in particular to those wishing to develop an interest in the field.

1: Introduction

The role of surgery in rheumatoid and certain broadly related diseases has changed enormously in recent years. Previously, procedures generally were of a salvage nature to try to prevent total collapse of the patient. In treating rheumatoid disease there was a fear of the possible effects of trauma – of increasing activity or of reactivating the disease – and so many rheumatologists were afraid to risk any form of surgery except as a last resort. In fact, in 1952, one of the authors proposed the use of electromyography, using needle electrodes, to study possible changes in the small muscles of the hand in relation to hand deformity; his rheumatologist colleagues considered it to be too dangerous, since it could possibly worsen the patient's condition.

Meanwhile, the concept of surgical removal of diseased synovium as a means of changing the progress of the disease at that particular site was becoming accepted. The realization that such a form of treatment could be practised with benefit, even in active disease, changed the whole concept of the management of at least classical rheumatoid diseases. Fortunately, the advent of surgery coincided with the introduction of several more potent forms of medical therapy such as gold, steroids, etc. Thus a more dynamic treatment of a depressing chronic disease became possible and enthusiasm accordingly increased. As so often happens, wild claims were made, not only for synovectomy but also for treatment with steroids; they were the revolutionary, new, long sought after cures. Some surgeons even took to synovectomy in rheumatoid disease with the confident attitude implied, and sometimes even spoken, that surgery alone could cure the disease. (Some physicians made similar claims for steroids – for a time.) The idea was that early synovectomy cured the disease in the joint so treated. Hence all that was required was to remove the synovium and thus the disease from all affected joints; the patients would be cured and rheumatologists no longer needed. But that was before the recurrences appeared, and now there are people who consider synovectomy of little or no value.

The introduction of gold follows almost the same pattern; there was great enthusiasm, then trials indicated that it had little effect and it was used much less. The wise rheumatologist, however, recognized in gold a valuable treatment and persisted in its use, and more recently it has once again been accepted but in a better perspective. The same is true for synovectomy; it will continue as a valuable form of treatment but with a much more careful selection of cases.

The introduction of early synovectomy was paralleled by the development of prosthetic joint replacements. Mechanically efficient hip prostheses have become such a boon to many patients with hip diseases that other joints were being and are being developed, such as finger joints. Again these were used with great enthusiasm to replace damaged interphalangeal and metacarpophalangeal joints, and again without proper care and selection of cases. Once again a more rational approach has developed as a result of problems in their use. The decision on whether to use them is usually now much more carefully analysed.

The important point that must be appreciated is that although rheumatoid arthritis is a commonly accepted term it is not just arthritis but a generalized disease affecting, in one way or another, virtually all the tissues of the body; and this is true of virtually all the related conditions.

In some conditions where surgery offers the best chance of success in treatment, it is proper that care should rest solely with the surgeon. For most of the rheumatological and related conditions, however, surgery can never be more than one form of therapy among several; effective at the proper time of the disease progression and in the proper patient. Rarely in a properly managed patient will surgery be used without concurrent medical therapy. Thus patients should be treated by the surgeon only under the general management of the physician. The physician should know what surgery might achieve, as he should know what each of his other forms of therapy has to offer. Conversely, the surgeon who includes himself in the treatment of rheumatoid diseases should understand at least something of the disease and ideally should work in close co-operation not only with the physician in charge of the case but also with the other therapists administering treatment. The closer the liaison which can be achieved the better will be the end result of therapy. For both the surgical authors of this book, planning of surgical treatment is usually decided at a joint clinic with the physician in charge.

Just as the selection of cases for surgery presents many problems in certain of the rheumatoid diseases, so in many cases does the surgical treatment. There are situations where a single operation is all that is required, but in many other cases surgery is being used as one facet in the treatment of a generalized disease process. As an example in the hand, to put in a prosthetic metacarpophalangeal joint is a simple technical exercise, but how the joint is to be used effectively is another matter. The patient may not have the will to use the hand postoperatively and every rheumatologist knows among his patients the women 'who have good husbands who do everything for them'. Such patients will have cosmetically satisfactory painless joints but the hands will not be used!

Many patients will have a series of inter-related problems affecting several joints and tendon systems, perhaps with arteritis of the digital arteries as well. A careful assessment of priorities thus becomes important. For instance, there is no point in performing a metacarpophalangeal joint replacement where there may be difficult muscular control of the joints owing to bulky tenosynovitis or even tendon rupture. If the fingers cannot be extended because the flexor tenosynovial bulk is too great to run through the fibrous flexor sheaths, then the metacarpophalangeal joints will not function even to the effective level expected of a prosthetic joint. Thus the tendons need to be cleared first before the joints are touched.

It is this type of problem which necessitates a careful

functional analysis of every case offered for surgery. Even the possible future progress of the disease must be considered. It is not reasonable to use a palmaris longus tendon to graft a ruptured extensor digiti minimi in a patient with grossly disorganized tendons of a more important nature which may at some time need that graft; simpler methods of repair will often suffice, leaving the spare parts for more vital possible needs.

Perhaps one of the most important considerations in such a form of treatment is to take the patient into the clinician's confidence. Most reasonably intelligent patients know that there is no cure for their disease but that with help they will probably not become a hopeless wreck. Patients are therefore often very perceptive about their own problems and, given reasonable facts, can often play a major part, not only in planning a surgical programme but in assisting the surgeon in the postoperative reactivation. The patient who knows the facts does not usually expect too much and any gain brings gratitude; the patient who does not know the facts expects a cure, and if this is not forthcoming then the surgeon is considered to have failed.

The surgical treatment of many of these conditions thus does not call for simple, stereotyped procedures. Each patient must be considered on merit and procedures planned for that individual patient, often in sequence. In conditions subject to so much variation in natural history – as, for instance, rheumatoid disease – many variations in surgical treatment are called for, though the principles remain the same. Furthermore, the surgical procedures are often of recent development and therefore quite different techniques may be practised by different surgeons to produce a similar end-result. In hand surgery, for instance, the surgeon's initial training – whether in orthopaedics or plastic surgery – may influence his surgical approaches to some extent. When it is remembered that many of the surgical procedures have been developed in the last 20 years, time has not yet allowed consolidation of techniques to a stereotyped pattern.

It will be obvious from this book that there are commonly two or more ways of solving the same problem. We have been heavily committed to developing hand surgery, in rheumatoid disease in particular, and have thus pursued to some extent parallel courses, developing our own ideas for solving a particular problem. We consider that in joining together to produce a common system of surgical procedures our different approaches should be illustrated rather than entirely resolved to a single technique. By so doing we believe that the flexibility of mind which is always necessary in the successful treatment of such conditions presenting such an enormous variation in natural history can be emphasized.

Surgical procedures in the various rheumatic or arthritic conditions are not necessarily specific for any individual disease. Operations are generally not designed to cure a particular disease process but rather to remove pathological material, to correct anatomical disorganization where that is possible, or to repair a disorganized anatomical situation to improve its current function. As a result, many of the surgical procedures are common to several different disease processes. Examples of this can readily be given. Synovectomy of a digital joint can be practised with good effect in both rheumatoid or psoriatic arthropathy. In rheumatoid disease there is usually bulky synovium, whereas in psoriatic arthropathy the synovium is often very thin with much secondary bony activity so that it is not unreasonable to doubt the value of synovectomy. Nevertheless, essentially the same operation on very different pathological synovium can often bring at least a few years of improvement and relief. Arthropathies of many kinds can lead to essentially similar destruction of joints, therefore it is sometimes of relatively little importance whether the bone changes are caused by rheumatoid arthritis, psoriatic arthritis, or osteoarthrosis of the region: if, for instance, the trapezium becomes grossly disorganized and painful an operation has to be done and probably the same operation regardless of the disease process. Hence it is our intention to illustrate rheumatoid disease as the prime need for the various operative procedures and to illustrate other conditions as much as is considered necessary within the confines of a book of reasonable size.

2: The principles of surgery in rheumatoid disease

Rheumatoid disease (or arthritis) is a generalized disease process and as such affects most tissues of the body to a greater or lesser extent. The most obvious feature is an inflammatory reaction affecting synovial membranes. As the most dramatic appearances tend to be in the joints, the term arthritis has become accepted. However, the other synovial membranes, tenosynovium, and bursae are also affected. In the hand, the diseased tenosynovium probably plays virtually as great a part in the destructive effects of the disease as do the diseased joints; this aspect is underestimated by many clinicians, largely through lack of appreciation of the amount of trouble in the palm under the thick palmar fascia, which makes examination difficult.

The natural history of the disease is highly variable; large numbers of people are affected but only a small proportion of these severely so. As a rough estimate, some 50 per cent of patients may be left with little or no disability, though some 10 per cent will have major physical incapacity. Of this last group, many can be given considerable help by what might be called salvage surgery, so allowing them to do a great deal for themselves. Few should become totally crippled with good modern medicine and good surgical support, particularly in the case of the patient with the will to cope with a sometimes ghastly disability.

It is a disease affecting mainly females, with estimates of 6 per cent of the female population compared with 2 per cent of males. It is often said to be a disease primarily of Europeans and European stock, being much less common elsewhere; but this is probably spurious. The apparent variation in incidence no doubt reflects the number of doctors knowing the treatability of the disease and, of course, the life expectancy in the community. Earlier death reduces the number of severe long-term cases seen.

The onset and course may be in short, sharp bursts (often separated as palindromic arthritis), episodic or persistent. In the episodic form the patient may have several attacks lasting some months, with apparent full remission for periods of years before complete remission or eventual deterioration to the chronic or persistent form. The chronic form also follows an undulent course but the periods of remission are relative; the disease persists but at a reduced level. Even in the persistent case the disease can become generally burnt out, or a joint showing marked if variable activity for many years can become burnt out, though the condition persists elsewhere. The joints so relieved then remain with post-rheumatoid osteoarthrosis, and the related soft tissue deformity can be treated as such.

Just as the onset and course is highly variable, so is the difficulty of prognosticating. Even a severe onset does not necessarily mean a hopeless future; apparent spontaneous recovery can occur even after severe illness of acute onset, possibly leaving physical ravages of the period of activity as a legacy.

With no completely effective cure for the disease, treatment is designed to reduce the inflammatory reaction, to lessen its effects during the active phase of the disease and to try to produce or accelerate the onset and rate of a recessive or healing phase. Surgery can sometimes play a useful part in support of medical therapy in the active phase of the disease and in an attempt to limit mechanical disorganization at a reasonably early stage. If the disease process can be controlled and mechanical damage limited then the patient is left with that physical damage which cannot repair naturally plus such extra degenerative problems as might arise later from living with a physical disability, e.g. the greater risk of osteoarthrosis, increased instability and abnormal function – here surgery can be of immense value.

In a condition with so much variation in presentation and course, assessment of the role that surgery can play also presents many difficulties. It must necessarily depend upon the individual case, its current presentation and expected history. This last consideration is extremely difficult to assess and decisions must depend largely on the clinician's experience, assisted by such evidence as has been accumulated from studies on the general history of the disease; in this case, on the hand. Such studies can be very valuable but can only be generalizations produced from the cases considered. The general picture may well be very different from the particular patient under consideration.

Nevertheless, certain deductions can be made and Kay's (1971) work on the history of the disease in the unoperated hand is of great value. She has shown a close parallel between the progress of the disease in the hand and our own studies in normal hand function. The likelihood of the disease appearing and, in particular, persisting is by far greatest in those components of the hand that cannot be rested. For example, if there is to be movement in a finger at all, there must be activity at its metacarpophalangeal joint. The interphalangeal joints need hardly be used, particularly in a painful hand; activity tends to be reduced to a precision-type grip, limiting movement to the digital metacarpophalangeal and the thumb carpo-metacarpal joints. In Kay's study the metacarpophalangeal joints are more likely to be affected than the interphalangeal joints, and the disease is more likely to persist there; whereas the interphalangeal joints, which can be rested, commonly recover. Similarly, if the fingers are to be used then the teno-synovium – particularly of the flexor tendons – must be at risk, with the index and middle fingers more vulnerable than the ring and little fingers. Thus an expectancy of progress in certain zones of the hand, if the disease should persist is possible, as is an indication of where help is likely to be needed and conversely where it is generally safe to observe and await developments.

Treatment of the disease obviously varies enormously with its severity and the necessity of using the more potent drugs, which are more likely to have unpleasant side effects. For many patients, mild anti-inflammatory drugs such as aspirin and phenylbutazone are sufficient if the disease is also mild, or in a quiescent state in a more severe case. In more severe and active phases, gold, chloroquin, steroids, penicillamine and immuno-suppressives might be required, either singly or in combination. It is generally preferable to use surgery in a less active phase of the disease wherever possible, but active disease is by no means a contraindication if surgery becomes necessary. For instance, synovectomy in a seropositive case of high activity (high erythrocyte sedimentation rate, etc.) is unlikely to succeed for long, unlike the excellent results usually obtained in less active disease with persistent bulky synovium. The more active the disease the greater the likelihood of recurrence after syno-vectomy. Thus the decision of which drugs to use and when – knowing that none are truly curative and, since this is a chronic disease, may have to be used over long periods, with possible severe side effects – presents the physician with difficult decisions. Also, since surgery is not curative but in certain phases of treatment can be highly valuable, there comes the equally difficult decision of when and what should be done or, preferably, be recommended to the patient. The decision must be the physicians, but a surgeon experienced in the field may know the vicissitudes of the disease as well as his physician colleague; joint consultation becomes immensely valuable. The surgeon has one advantage over the physician; he has the chance of comparing the clinical picture with the condition found under the skin at operation. We believe very strongly that joint consultation is essential whenever surgery is contemplated even if the physician's contemplation is initially only tentative. The physician in his consideration of the disease commonly does not see the whole physical picture, because of his concentration on the systemic disease process, whereas the surgeon may see the physical problems in isolation from the disease.

At the initial assessment for surgery, one important possibility should be considered – digital arteritis, which may lead to partial or virtually total obliteration of the lumen of the artery. It is not too difficult with practice to feel a digital pulse, but if in doubt various other tests are available such as use of a Doppler machine. In any case, care must be taken with the arteries, particularly in rheumatoid disease, as minor amounts of arteritis are not clinically estimable.

As with any other inflammatory reaction, rest is a valuable form of therapy but it inevitably leads to the musculo-skeletal changes arising from simple disuse. This situation is aggravated by the natural reflex inhibition to movement, particularly in those joints where the muscular movement materially increases intra-articular pressure on bulky synovium; the knees and the metacarpophalangeal joints of the hand are the most obvious examples of this. Muscular contraction of the quadriceps in the case of the knee and the muscles entering the extensor expansion over the metacarpophalangeal joints of the hand increases the already raised joint pressure due to the disease and there is the tendency for reflex inhibition of such muscles. In the hand, the interossei often become particularly affected by the disease process in this way, with loss or reduction of their normal very important control over the metacarpophalangeal joints, which become more unstable. In the end this can lead to considerable disuse atrophy of the muscles and, owing to synovial bulk stretching articular and periarticular soft tissues, a loss of the normal control of the joints. The ulnar drift is a dramatic end-result of this process but, far more important and

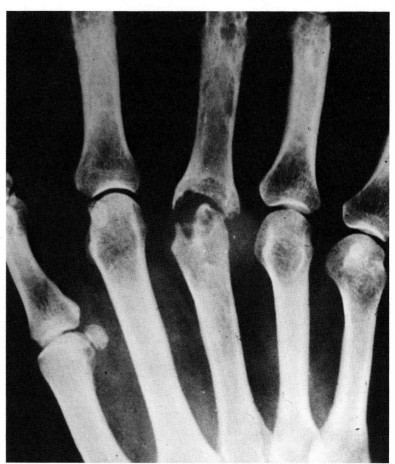

2.1

less appreciated, so is the volar subluxation and eventual dislocation.

If the patient fights against the disease and uses the hand, then the inflammatory reaction in the joints, including synovial bulk and intra-articular pressure, will be increased. Owing to the work, strength may be maintained in the articular and periarticular tissues, but with the expense of bone erosion and destruction. The patient who protects her hand and does nothing to help herself may have much soft-tissue disorganization and deformity but the bone in relation to the joint may show no more than the osteoporosis of disuse and the joint cartilage may appear virtually normal. The patient who insists on activity may show little deformity other than swollen joints but severe bone destruction. The naturally produced so-called egg and cup arthroplasty, described by Vaughan–Jackson, appears to be due to this process; the distal end of the metacarpal becomes so eroded laterally that it collapses within the joint, leaving a small end (the egg) fitting into the eroded, hollowed phalangeal base. Radiologically the picture appears disastrous but function can be remarkably good (**Figure 2.1**).

The physical effect of the disease thus depends not only on its course and activity but also to an enormous extent on the attitude and activities of the patient. As surgery deals to a great extent with the physical situation of the patient in relation to the disease, these attitudes and activities are very important in not only what surgical treatment may be advised but also whether surgery should be advised at all.

Inevitably, any disease process has a profound effect on the patient as a whole; and a chronic, often painful condition such as rheumatoid disease with the possibility, always in the patient's mind, of being crippled and helpless can produce quite severe problems. These aggravate the natural psychosomatic characteristics of the patient. Many patients accept their condition with remarkable fortitude and show an ability to not only work through their disability but also actively co-operate with their medical advisors in therapy. Others cope only by demanding support from those around. Surgery can be of value for many patients with rheumatoid disease but the surgeon needs the patient's co-operation. In the latter group of patients, the co-operation may not be forthcoming, not only because of the lack of willpower but even more in some cases because of the knowledge that surgery may, if successful, mean an undesirable reduction in the need for support. It is just as important when considering surgery in rheumatoid disease to assess these psychological attitudes of the patient to the disease as it is to assess the disease processes themselves.

MacIndoe's dictum was that: 'it is not what the surgeon does to the hand that matters but what the patient does with it afterwards.' In view of the mental effects of a chronic painful disease, this aspect is particularly important; surgery on the wrong patient can be disastrous whereas the same operation on the right patient with an apparently comparable disease state might restore hand function and the ability to work.

Preparation of the patient for surgery is important in a disease which cannot be cured. It is essential to take the patient into the clinician's confidence and to explain what is likely to be achieved. If the patient thinks of an operation as a cure for the disease in the hand then disappointment will be inevitable. With explanation of what is being advised and stressing its limitations, the patient is likely to accept such improvements as are gained with gratitude and thus start the postoperative activity satisfactorily.

Many operations in rheumatoid hand disease are carried out on functionally disorganized hands and hence with joints operating over sometimes bizarre ranges and muscles equally ineffective. Many hundreds of prosthetic metacarpophalangeal joints must have been inserted under these conditions with little or no improvement in function, though the patient accepted the situation happily, having lost the preoperative pain. With proper preoperative mobilization in the physiotherapy department and an assurance that the components of the hand needing to be used postoperatively are functionally able to do so, the end-results might well have been far better. Surgery carried out in the rheumatoid hand without proper consideration of the whole picture of the disease process, the patient's attitude to the disease, proper preparation for the operation and follow-up therapy all mediate to produce unsatisfactory end-results and disillusion in a most valuable and rewarding field of surgery.

Related arthropathies

Rheumatoid disease is only one of many arthropathies where surgery can play a valuable role. Generally the patterns and problems associated with surgery are comparable even though the diseases themselves may show different manifestations. But this is not true of rheumatoid disease itself. It might be expected that in a true seropositive rheumatoid arthropathy or tenosynovitis the behaviour of the synovial pathology might be comparable, but this is far from true. One case will produce a thick bulky synovial mass whereas another, apparently similar clinically, will produce a comparable swelling made up of contained modified synovial fluid, sometimes with melon-seed or similar fibrinoid bodies, with relatively thin synovium. Both are, however, likely to produce disruption of surrounding tissues but the latter is more amenable to removal of fluid by needle and permit local hydrocortisone therapy. Where tendons are affected, some cases of synovitis may produce underlying tendon damage (more likely in the drier, fleshy form) whereas others may show little underlying tendon pathology. Sometimes quite small tenosynovial bulk may nevertheless lead to unexpected underlying tendon damage, whereas in other cases the synovial bulk will be considerable whilst the tendons beneath may nevertheless show a clean, glossy surface. We have also found that the mode of treatment can often produce characteristic appearance of the synovium at operation. For instance, gold therapy commonly produces fibrosis, giving the synovium a firm, drier character. Gold not infrequently leads to considerable fibrosis which can actually bind the tendon to surrounding structures, thus limiting tendon movement. Steroid therapy tends to produce a wet, soft synovium whereas penicillamine produces firm, sticky material often with a blood-stained exudate; this last type of synovium is difficult to clean from tendon or joint surface at synovectomy.

In view of the wide variety of synovial features even within seropositive rheumatoid disease, it is hardly surprising that there is enormous overlap in the gross joint pathology among the various inflammatory arthropathies. Some characteristic features can be recognized. For instance, the seronegative arthropathy often found in association with psoriasis – psoriatic arthropathy very commonly affects the terminal digital interphalangeal joints to a great extent, whereas mild effects only are seen in a small proportion of cases of seropositive rheumatoid disease. In psoriatic arthropathy great synovial bulk is unusual and the synovium may be very thin and may look almost normal macroscopically even where there is severe joint destruction. Joint destruction is very much a feature of psoriatic arthropathy and there may be periarticular bone overgrowth. This sequence of events often leads to considerable deformity of the fingers and joints, which stiffen in unacceptable positions (**Figure 1**, page 176).

Fixation of joints in unacceptable positions is also often a feature of juvenile arthropathy (Still's disease). Here the wrist often shows severe deformity (**Figure 2**, page 204).

Inevitably the ravages of the various inflammatory arthropathies lead, even with burnt-out disease, to a comparable situation of degenerative arthrosis or osteoarthrosis, which in these cases is often aggravated by instability of the joint. Thus, much of the treatment in the later stages of these diseases and pure osteoarthrosis may be virtually the same.

Surgical treatment

The surgical treatment will vary with the state of the disease. In many patients the hand may require surgical support at only

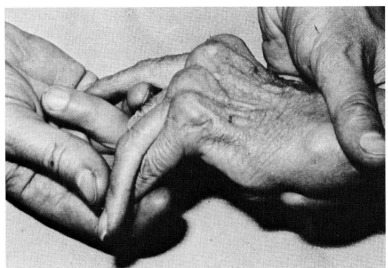

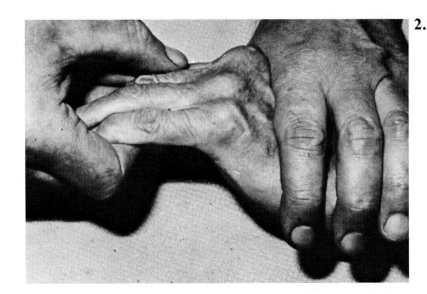

one site, as for instance a carpal-tunnel compression secondary to tenosynovitis or a single trigger finger. In others there may be, and in most persistent rheumatoid hands there usually is, a variety of sites at which surgery may be required or at least considered. Certainly in the more advanced cases there may be several sites or systems showing thick diseased synovium, joint destruction, or tendon rupture. In the case where there is an obvious single major lesion, the decision of what to do presents few problems other than whether to operate or to attempt treatment by other means.

In the more generally affected hand there may well be a state of multiple disorganization of the chain of joints. To operate on what at first sight appears to be the most obvious deformity – such as ulnar drifting, volar subluxing, or metacarpophalangeal joints – when there is thick flexor tenosynovium limiting digital extension and adaptedly shortened muscles controlling the system is illogical. Yet it is done so often, without proper consideration of the whole hand and the preparation of a planned sequence of treatment, that surgery in some quarters has fallen into disrepute. The problem is, then, not the failure of surgery but of the surgeon to understand normal hand function and its dysfunction secondary to rheumatoid disease. No one should operate on a rheumatoid hand, except for simple problems, without a proper consideration of the sequence of events leading to the clinical state and then only after assessing a sequence of functional priorities in the repair. As an example, in the case of the disorganized metacarpophalangeal joints quoted above the flexor tendons may need a synovectomy so as to allow the tendons to run freely into the digital fibrous flexor sheaths, thus allowing full digital extension and reducing much stress on the metacarpophalangeal joints. Then the hand should be treated by stretching of the contracted muscles and possibly exercising of these muscles so as to give maximum mobility and potential postoperative control of the hand. Only then should surgery be attempted on the metacarpophalangeal joints (**Figure 2.2**).

Many prosthetic metacarpophalangeal and other arthroplasties of these joints have been performed without proper preparation of the patient and the hand preoperatively with the eventual less than satisfactory result. This is unsatisfactory surgical treatment even though the surgical technique may be good. The value of treating the hand by surgery, not only in rheumatoid disease but in other fields as well, depends not so much on a scrupulous technique (this should be taken for granted) but on the clinical ability to pin-point the primary target for surgery in a possible sequence of events. Not infrequently an apparently useless hand with a multiplicity of problems can be given adequate function by a relatively simple procedure; the problem is to spot the correct procedure.

Conversely, as the disease is likely to produce a chain-reaction in which one deformity leads to another, it is important to define the changes early and accurately. The sequence can then often be interrupted and so prevent major deformity occurring later.

Surgical treatment can therefore be considered under the following headings:

1 Prophylactic.
2 Symptomatic.
3 Reconstructive.
4 Salvage.

Prophylactic treatment

Some years ago the idea was put forward that early synovectomy of a joint might remove the diseased synovium from it before damage was done to the surrounding structures and that the new replacement synovium, when it developed, might be normal. The advocates of the concept insisted that it must be done early and in any case before bone erosion appeared if it was to be successful. The difficulty immediately arose as to which joints of the many possibly affected should be so treated and what was meant by early. Longer-term studies have shown that there is a high recurrence rate (some 60 per cent in a 5-year follow-up) and that this is greater and more rapid in cases with more-active disease. Furthermore, as shown by Kay's work, many joints will recover either by natural remission or after medical treatment. Generally it can now be accepted that early synovectomy is sometimes valuable, particularly in those sites where the disease is most likely to persist – for instance, the metacarpophalangeal joints – and in those cases where reasonable medical treatment has not cleared the bulk of synovium as the disease has subsided. Removal of the bulk in a moderately controlled case commonly give good results. The radiographic use of erosions as an index of effectiveness has received far too much prominence. However, this relies on interpreting a picture, not the patient's function, and hence should not be given too much credence. Erosions may continue to exist or even to grow at a reduced rate, but most patients show much improved function and reduced pain after synovectomy, at least for several years. We are dealing with the surgical treatment of rheumatoid disease – not with cure, but with clinical improvement, reduction of pain and mechanical limitation of function, and the reclamation of those patients who have already become disabled. If the erosions are thoroughly cleaned out and the synovectomy reasonably effectively done then, if the disease can be controlled medically, the operation will be successful. The dividing line between early and later synovectomy has been deliberately blurred in these statements. The object of this is to stress that although early synovectomy is to be preferred in cases where it appears advisable, the idea that it must be done before erosions appear, or the operation will be useless, is quite erroneous, though too commonly believed.

Symptomatic treatment

The object of prophylaxis is to prevent or limit further synovial activity in the operated site and also to prevent possible disruption of surrounding tissues. Symptomatic treatment affects conditions in which the synovitis is producing secondary effects in surrounding local structures and there may be danger of initiating a chain-reaction of more extensive disruption. Flexor tenosynovectomy (or even simple carpal-tunnel decompression) may be performed for carpal-tunnel compression of the median nerve (many carpal-tunnel compressions are associated with non-specific or rheumatoid tenosynovitis). A trigger finger if not cleared, particularly in rheumatoid disease, may rapidly lead to fixed flexion deformity of the interphalangeal joints' collateral ligaments, thus aggravating any tendency to volar subluxation. Thickened synovium being pulled through retinaculi not only causes friction and hence tendency to volar subluxation. Thickened synovium being pulled through reticuli not only causes friction and hence aggravation of the tenosynovitis but also much increased pressure at the end of the synovial sheath. This occurs at the proximal end of the digital sheath as the fingers are extended, pulling such synovium and contained fluid as will go into the fibrous flexor sheath of the fingers but leaving a mass behind under pressure (**Figure 5.2**, page 55); at the distal end of the palmar synovial bursa as tendons are pulled through the carpal tunnel and, on the dorsum of the hand, at the distal end of the extensor tenosynovial sheaths as the tendons are pulled through the extensor fibro-osseous compartment. Thus there is likely damage to tendons beneath any synovial sheath under load but the greatest risk to tendons is in these three sites, with the possibility of rupture (**Figure 5.1**, page 55). Occasionally, tendons may be damaged by bone spicules secondary to bone erosion, but this is uncommon, as also is damage from the hypermobile and deformed end of the ulna.

In addition to the tenosynovitis, removal of synovial bulk

from joints reduces stress on related structures and the risk of not only further damage to the joint, but in many cases of the initiation of a sequence of damage. As an example of local effects, bulky synovium in the metacarpophalangeal joints produces not only less-effective lubricant for the joint but also considerable pressure in surrounding structures; the capsule and collateral ligaments become stretched leading to volar subluxation; the extensor expansion is stretched, particularly at its weakest point to the radial side of the extensor tendon, leading to ulnar dislocation of the tendon and so producing ulnar drift and ineffective extensor control (**Figure 3.15**, page 25); back pressure on venous outflow channels from the bone leads to bone damage and erosions.

Relatively simple procedures at this stage can do a great deal to limit major disruption due to chain reactions. If these can be recognized and the procedures performed early enough the progress to deformity can be interrupted. In addition to those chain-reactions already mentioned, there are many more in the hand, for example:

1 Pain and swelling around the ulnar styloid leads to protective radial deviation of the wrist, which may become fixed.
2 Radial deviation of the wrist has been said to induce ulnar drift of the fingers or vice versa in a form of Z collapse. (It must be stressed, however, that this correlation is as yet not proven; the conditions are probably correlated but not mutually dependent problems.)
3 Volar subluxation of the digital metacarpophalangeal joints can lead to swan-neck deformity.
4 Dislocation ulnarwards of the extensor tendons may lead to uncontrolled ulnar drift and also, because of adaptive shortening of the interossei, to intrinsic snap and swan-neck deformity.
5 Synovial proliferation of the proximal interphalangeal joints can lead to stretching of the extensor tendon and boutonniere deformity.
6 Thumb carpometacarpal joint synovitis (among other causes) can lead to adduction of the metacarpal with compensatory radial deviation and instability of the thumb metacarpophalangeal joint.
7 Subluxation of the thumb metacarpophalangeal joint commonly leads to fixed hyperextension of the interphalangeal joint (the so-called Z deformity). This, in turn, can lead to avulsion of the flexor tendon, especially if it has been weakened by synovitis.
8 The establishment of ulnar drift of one finger can precipitate the condition in all.

This list is not intended to be exhaustive but merely to indicate the importance of early recognition of the local physical symptoms and signs secondary to rheumatoid synovitis; its simple surgical treatment can prevent disability and the need for reconstructive and salvage procedures later.

Reconstructive treatment

Once deformity has occurred then reconstruction is obviously a much more extensive problem, particularly as the deformity is often long-standing before the patient is referred to the surgeon. Muscles show gross adaptive shortening which makes the dynamic control of the postoperative hand difficult, whilst ligaments are often stretched with collagen change and hence not likely to be effectively repaired by simple anatomical tightening. Ruptured tendons can rarely be repaired directly, because of the necrosis that usually occurs before rupture. Usually, reconstructive surgery requires a sequence of operations in a carefully worked out plan for the best results. Operative treatments required include:

1 Repair of flexor and extensor tendons by grafts or tendon-lengthening procedures.
2 Correction of swan-neck deformity.
3 Correction of boutonnière deformity.
4 Ulnar styloidectomy for subluxing, hypermobile ulnar head and for pronation-supination pain or disability.
5 Correction of hypermobile, painful wrist and carpal joints by synovectomy and postoperative external fixation to allow some stiffening.
6 Correction of ulnar drift and subluxation of the metacarpophalangeal joints.
7 Correction of abductor deformity of the little finger by reconstruction of ligaments and muscle realignment.
8 Correction of thumb adduction deformity due to carpometacarpal joint damage.

Salvage treatment

1 Excision arthroplasty.
2 Interposition arthroplasty.
3 Arthrodesis.

Established deformities are all too often seen as the end result of a chain-reaction, in which no attempt has been made to interrupt the inevitable progress to deformity. To restore some function to hands requires procedures which are destructive and irrevocable.

Subluxation of the metacarpophalangeal joints often cannot be corrected without excision of the head of the metacarpal.

Having established a correction, the problem is to maintain it. Several procedures are recorded for excision arthroplasty by different authors, but in many cases it becomes necessary to use the principles of interposition arthroplasty, in which either a malleable or rigid strut is inserted between the bone ends to maintain the alignment, either temporarily or permanently.

Arthrodesis
This is indicated for gross destructive changes with secondary deformities in digital joints, and also in the wrist joint. The first metacarpophalangeal joint is a common site for arthrodesis, and the terminal joint of the thumb in both adult and juvenile patients with rheumatism often becomes unstable. The proximal interphalangeal joint requires fusion when the joint surfaces are destroyed, and the digit is in fixed extension or unstable. The terminal joints of the fingers are often affected in psoriatic arthritis; a characteristic feature is gross destructive changes in the bone ends. Arthrodesis of the wrist becomes necessary in those patients who have had an insidious medial shift (glissement carpien), as in juvenile patients. Instability with deformity is an indication for fusion, in both juveniles and adults.

Just as the metacarpophalangeal joint of the fingers and the carpometacarpal joint of the thumb are the ones which cannot be rested and hence are more likely to show persistent disease, so also there are the joints which need if possible to be retained in activity. Hence, in a deformed or unstable finger interphalangeal arthrodesis in a good functional position can be most valuable and give excellent results, often converting a virtually useless hand into a most effective instrument; the metacarpophalangeal joint should, however, work effectively. In the thumb, arthrodesis of either or both interphalangeal and metacarpophalangeal joints can be valuable so long as the carpometacarpal joint functions well. In the thumb, however, so long as there is good functional control over the metacarpophalangeal joints – as is often the case in osteoarthrosis of the carpometacarpal region – this joint can be fixed, possibly allowing increased mobility of the metacarpophalangeal joint to give adequate thumb activity.

3: Assessment for hand surgery

General assessment

The manifestations of rheumatoid and the related diseases are protean and can concern many disciplines.

The rheumatologist will be a physician and thus able to consider the medical aspects of the general assessment. He will maintain overall control of the patient and co-ordinate the different specialists that are needed occasionally in the treatment of any patient.

Joint clinics are highly desirable, as emphasized previously, so that the different aspects of the patient's illness can be discussed. Often surgical treatment will be contraindicated even when the hand appears in need of possible surgical intervention, because of the more necessary primary medical care. The timing of surgery in the overall treatment programme can be discussed. Having come to the conclusion that the time is optimal for surgery, there may be priorities in the form or site of treatment. For instance, surgery for a foot or knee may be more urgent than for the hand or vice versa. These priorities need to be discussed between rheumatologist and surgeon.

Before any form of surgery there must be an effective general medical assessment which will include erythrocyte sedimentation rate and serum tests. General examination should include the eyes, nervous system, chest, heart and abdomen, including

the genitourinary tract. Arthritis is often associated with a wide variety of diseases of other systems of the body such as ulcerative colitis, psoriasis and various infections, particularly gonococcal, etc. Amyloidosis is not uncommon as a terminal feature of rheumatoid disease.

Supplementary evidence of the condition can be provided by radiography and the neck and chest are areas which should be routinely X-rayed apart from the specific investigations. It is particularly important that routine chest and neck radiographs are taken before surgery; it is not uncommon to see severe destructive changes and instability in the cervical vertebral joints. It is our practice to X-ray the necks of all patients before surgery (**Figure 3.1**), noting particularly the movement between the anterior arch of the atlas and the odontoid peg in flexion. Instability of the neck obviously presents problems in anaesthesia, particularly if intubation is considered.

One of us (SHH) uses axillary blocks for anaesthesia routinely in rheumatic patients. This reduces the risks and avoids the immediate pain and discomfort after a hand operation, as long-acting regional anaesthesia continues for many hours after the operation.

It is not so common now to see a patient on high steroid

3.1a

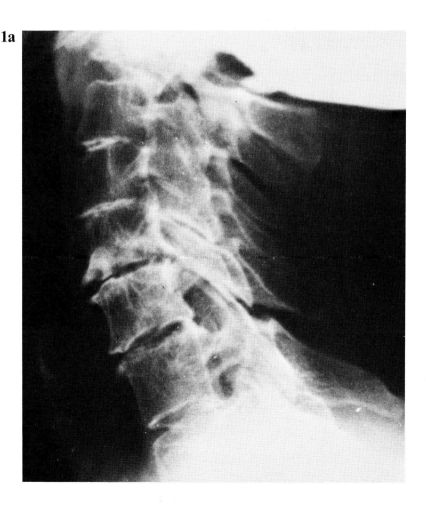

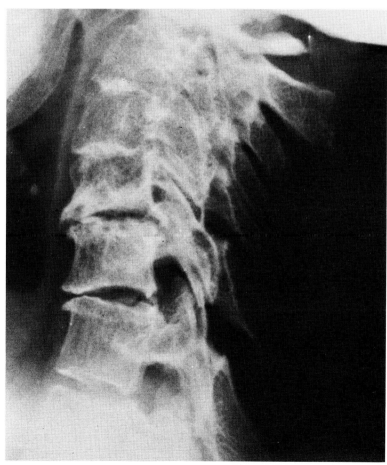

3.1b

	RIGHT		LEFT	
	F.D.	E.D.	F.D.	E.D.
INDEX				
MIDDLE				
RING				
LITTLE				
F.D.-FLEXOR DEFICIT-E.D.-EXTENSOR				

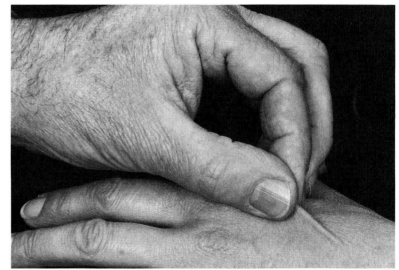

intake, but evidence of having taken these drugs can be seen in the fragility of the superficial blood vessels, which often present as bruising on the dorsum of the hand and in the thin atrophic skin. Such patients may be slow to heal and it is desirable in those patients taking prednisolone to defer surgical treatment until the intake is reduced to 7.5 mg daily if possible. In any case it is important to record if the patient has been taking steroids, even in the previous 2 years or so, and to warn the anaesthetist. Even as long as 2 years after steroid therapy it is advisable to give an intravenous steroid supplement at the time of operation to prevent the risk of postoperative 'steroid shock', a problem which anyone considering surgery in a patient taking steroids must be aware of; its effect can be very disturbing on both patient and medical and nursing staff.

Rheumatoid vasculitis may materially affect the blood supply of a limb and a manifestation of this endothelial proliferation in the small blood vessels may be seen as pinpoint areas of vasculitis around the nail.

Just as the whole body should be examined before considering the hand, so should the rest of the limb, shoulder, elbow and forearm, for the hand can usually only be effective on an effective limb.

Hand assessment

Progressive functional disability in the rheumatic patient can be so insidious that disability is not recognized until it is established. An assessment of hand function therefore requires careful analysis, and should be done by one trained in hand function and functional anatomy. The basic actions of pinch and grip are apparent, but their anatomical interpretation requires detailed study. The anatomy included in normal function should be known, as this forms the basis for understanding the alteration in function which occurs when anatomy is distorted either by injury or disease. It is just as important to know what a patient cannot do as what she can.

The occupational therapist should attend the joint clinics and do a hand assessment on all new patients. A form should be compiled on which results of tests carried out to assess the patient's capability to perform basic functions are noted. The functions will come under the two main headings of grip and pinch. Grip will be sub-divided into power grip and hook grip. Pinch is sub-divided into fine pinch, power pinch and key pinch. A proforma in current practice in one of our clinics (SHH) can be seen on page 19.

These tests are followed by more-advanced assessment in which strength, sensory function, and stereognosis is interpreted and recorded. All these tests will determine the patient's ability to perform their normal domestic duties, with or without difficulty, and will also determine a patient's ability to perform his job. Photographs of the hand should be taken, and these should conform to a standard available at all clinics (page 20).

Simple measurement of finger range should be done in all cases, and recorded on a die stamp table (top left). These records not only illustrate the flexor and extensor deficit at the time of the first visit, but are a useful method of assessing either progress or regression of the disease in the hand.

Examination of the hand

Firstly, the skin should be examined (**Figure 3.2**). It may be hot and sweating, particularly in the active phase of the disease.

The skin may be thin and atrophic from disuse, or when the patient is on a steroid drug; then bruising may be seen on the dorsum of the hand or the forearm. Steroid treatment may be associated with a characteristic facial appearance.

Panel 1

HAND ASSESSMENT **1**

NAME: DATE:
ADDRESS: OCCUPATION:

NOTES No: CONSULTANT:
AGE:
DOMINANT HAND: DEFORMITIES:

1. ASSESSMENT OF FUNCTION:

(a) Pinch	
(i) Precision pinch (tip-to-tip)	Pencil writing name:
	Using tweezers
	Picking up a pin
(ii) Lateral pinch (key pinch)	Holding a plate
	Turning key in lock
	Pulling away a postcard
(iii) Power pinch	Pulling string
	Plucking putty
	Needle & thread
	Peg
(iv) Tripod pinch	Picking up draughts
	Screw-top lid
	Tap
	Dowelling - various
	Putting plug in socket

COMMENTS:

(b) Grip	
(i) Small-tool grip	Screwdriver, knife or fork
(ii) Cylinder grip	Holding hammer/chisel
(iii) Hook Grip	Lifting hand of watering can/kettle

Panel 2

HAND ASSESSMENT: **2**
NAME:
NOTES NO:

(b) Grip (Continued) (iv) Span	Opening scissors
	Holding large ball
	Lifting can from above

COMMENTS:

(c) Release	Throwing a ball
(d) Co-ordination	Carrying full glass of water
(e) Strength	Lifting 12 lb box with both hands
(f) Sensory function	Localisation
(g) Stereognosis	Cotton wool
	Key
	Coin
	Safety Pin
	Foam Square
	Wood Square
	Hot
	Cold
(h) Pronation and supination of wrist	

COMMENTS:

2. PROBLEMS IN ADL:

(a) Dressing	Buttons
	Zips
	Shoelaces

Panel 3

HAND ASSESSMENT: **3**
NAME:
NOTES NO:

2. (b) Washing	Taps.
	Handling soap, toothbrush etc.
(c) Eating	Cutlery
	Holding cup to drink
	Pouring liquids
	Feeding

COMMENTS:

3. LIMITATIONS RELATED TO WORK:

(a) Writing	
(b) Handling money	
(c) Particular problems	

COMMENTS:

4.

ELABORATION OF ASSESSMENT FOR PINCH	Index	Middle	Ring	Little
(a) Rubber				
(b) Metal nut				
(c) Clothes peg (open and close)				
(d) Screw				
(e) Large rubber band				
(f) Peg-board dowel				
(g) Safety pin (open and close)				
(h) Paper clip				
(i) Nail				
(j) Drawing pin				
(k) Small rubber band				
(l) 2p coin				

Panel 4

4

4. ELABORATION OF ASSESSMENT FOR PINCH. (Continued)

	Index	Middle	Ring	Little
(m) 1p coin				
(n) ½p coin				
(o) Panel pin				
(p) Pin				
(q) Needle				
(r) Pass threaded needle through paper and pull through				

SUMMARY:

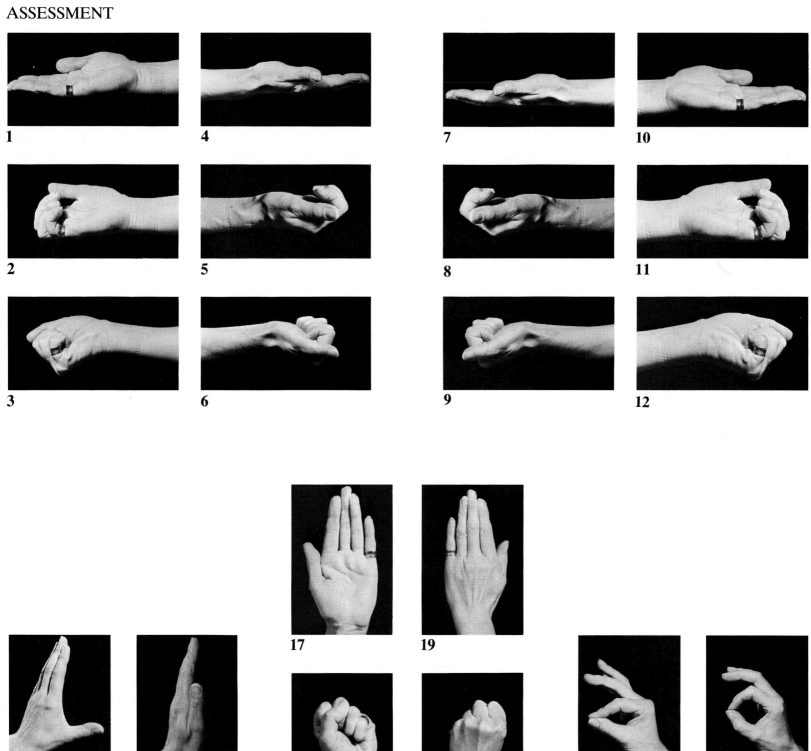

1 **4** **7** **10**

2 **5** **8** **11**

3 **6** **9** **12**

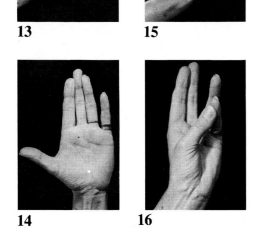

13 **15**

14 **16**

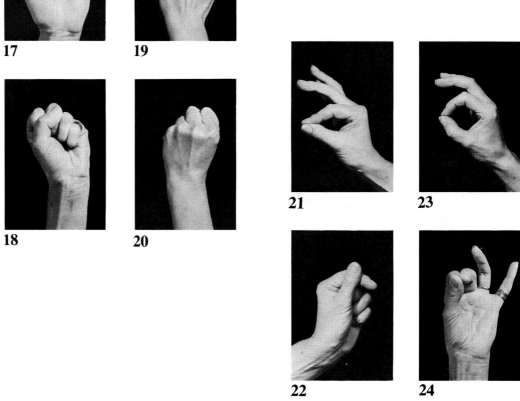

17 **19**

18 **20**

21 **23**

22 **24**

3.3

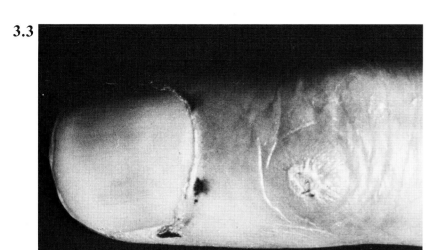

3.4

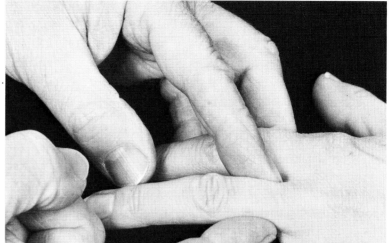

3.5

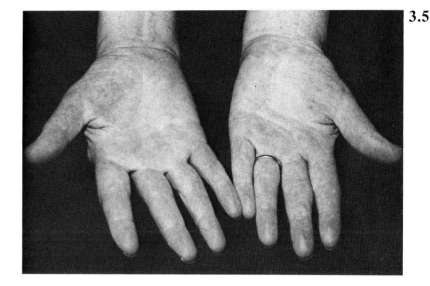

Pinpoint ulceration around the nail bed is an indication of vasculitis (**Figure 3.3**). If this is present the digital arteries should be examined for patency by a direct pulse (**Figure 3.4**) or by such methods as a Dopplermeter.

Brown pigmentation or pitting of the nail is often associated with psoriatic arthritis. Beau's lines, which are transverse grooves in the nail, are an indication of recent illness.

Erythema of the hypothenar and sometimes the thenar eminence is not uncommonly seen in rheumatic patients, but it is not necessarily evidence of liver deficiency (**Figure 3.5**). In cold weather, many patients show evidence of poor circulation, similar to the cyanosis seen in Raynaud's disease. If ulceration in the fingers is associated with adherent skin on the dorsum then scleroderma should be considered.

Secondly, examination of the deep structures affected in the hand should commence proximally and proceed distally. Ranges and freedom of movement of the shoulder and elbow joint will have been recorded in the general examination.

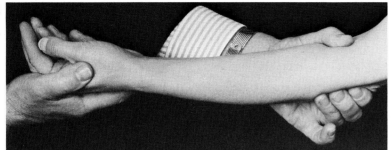

3.6a

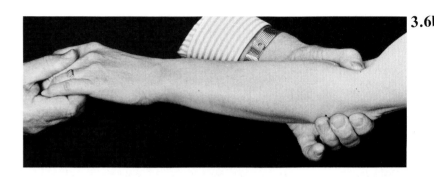

3.6b

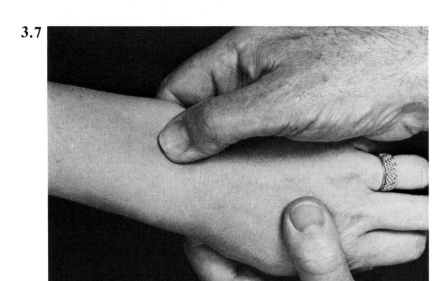

3.7

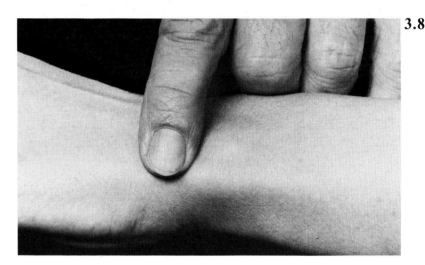

3.8

Radio-ulnar joints

Movement of the radio-ulnar joints must now be examined with pronation and supination. Any blocking of movement is recorded, as is any associated pain together with the position in which it is felt. If there is evidence of mechanical disturbance examination of those movements should be carried out initially with the fingers over the radial head (**Figure 3.6**) and then over the distal end of the ulna. Hence it is usually possible to diagnose whether disability is associated with the proximal or distal joints, or possibly both.

Proliferation of synovial tissue is particularly common in the distal radio-ulnar joint, which may extrude and form a pouch around the ulnar styloid. This may be a painful swelling and can lead to protective and eventually fixed deviation of the wrist. In the more advanced cases, the radio-ulnar ligament (triangular fibrocartilage) ruptures and the head is free to subluxate dorsally in pronation, producing mobility and pain. Pressure on the ulnar head in the prone position is followed by a rebound, and this is called the 'ping-pong' sign (**Figure 3.7**). The ulnar styloid is free to move dorsally in pronation due to the extensor carpi ulnaris tendon which lies over the dorsum of the ulna in supination, being carried on to the border of the ulna in pronation (**Figure 3.8**). This is a normal movement of the tendon and not, as is often supposed, secondary to rheumatoid arthritis of the joint.

The ulnar head, when mobile and distorted, can rub against the lower end of the radius producing a scalloped appearance on a radiograph. This condition may be painful, necessitating excision of the ulnar head.

3.9a

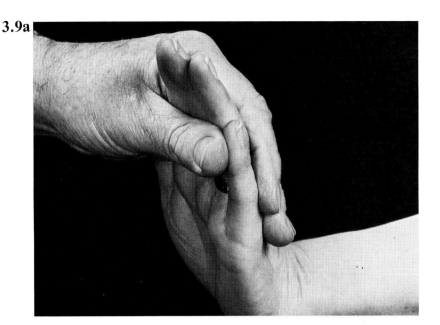

3.9b

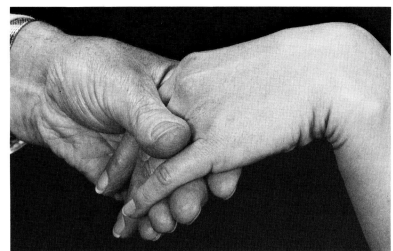

.10a

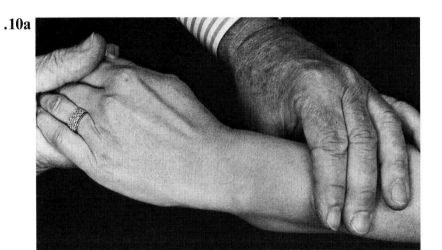

3.10b

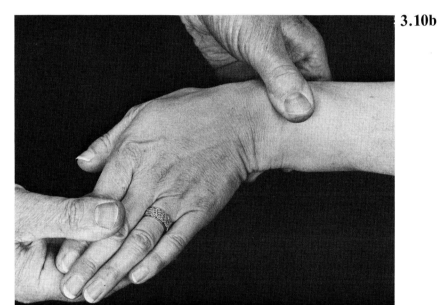

The wrist and carpal joints

Flexion and extension and particularly ulnar and radial deviation should be examined (**Figures 3.9** and **3.10**) whilst at the same time noting how the patient normally holds the hand. Passive examination of ulnar deviation should at first be done with great care as this movement may be painful and the patient may resist movement, so giving a false impression. A similar movement but giving pain over the radial border is characteristic of De Quervain's disease.

In seronegative juvenile chronic polyarthritis, swelling of the wrist and carpal joints with flexion deformity is often one of the earliest features. Gross destructive changes in the wrist can, however, occur both in juvenile and adult rheumatoid arthritis. The hand and carpus may subluxate volarwards or shift medially, in which case the deformity is called 'glissement carpien'. In both cases, once deformity is established, arthrodesis to produce stability may be required.

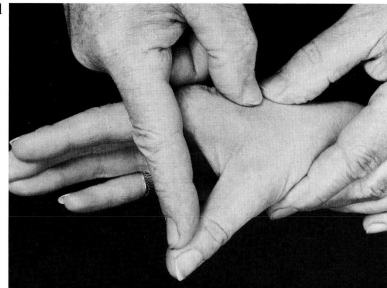

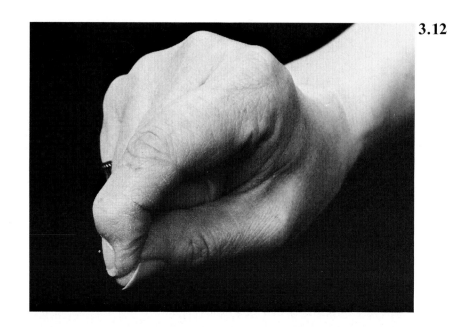

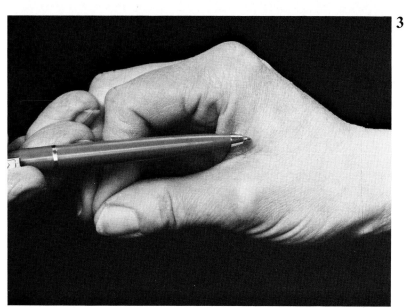

Carpometacarpal joint of the thumb

Destructive change in this joint is very common, not only in the inflammatory diseases but also as osteoarthrosis. It may be localized to the carpometacarpal joint alone, as may follow a Bennett's fracture, but more commonly it also affects the mid-carpal components at the thumb base. Major changes may occur at the joint after rheumatoid disease, with the tendency for the metacarpal bone to sublux off the trapezium. Even without this occurring there may be a tendency for the thumb to collapse towards the index finger, producing an adduction deformity either as a result of changed mechanics, or apparently held as a protection against pain. There may later be secondary shortening of the musculature in the web. The change in position of the metacarpal can lead to excessive strain on the medial collateral ligament of the first metacarpophalangeal joint, which may stretch or rupture and produce radial deviation (**Figure 3.11**).

This deformity alters the mechanism of pinch between the thumb and index fingers, from pulp-to-pulp opposition (**Figure 3.12**) to apposition (**Figure 3.13**). The index tends to pronate to withstand the pressure of the thumb and therefore needs a strongly acting first dorsal interroseous muscle (**Figure 3.14**) and the support of the middle finger.

3.15

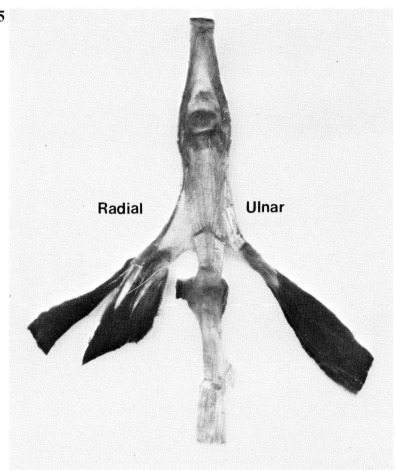

Radial   Ulnar

3.16

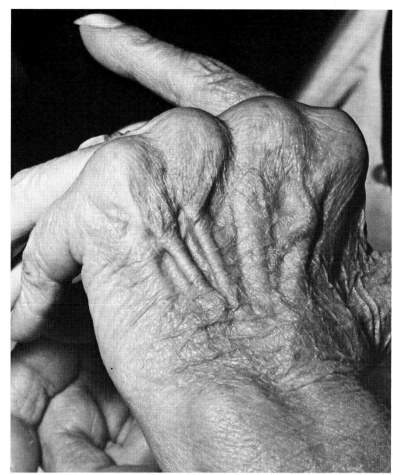

3.17

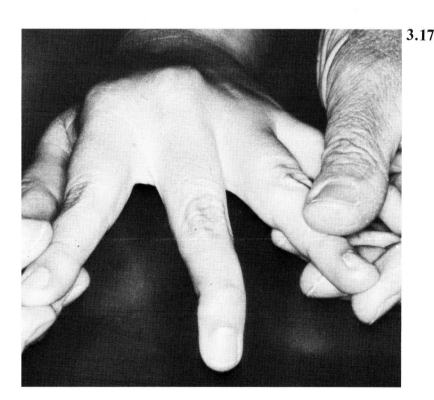

Thumb joints

The thumb metacarpophalangeal joint is nowhere near as important a joint as its digital counterpart; nevertheless, it may suffer severe disability. Not only may it become hypermobile in a radial direction but other changes may occur after synovitis. There may be severe stretching of the extensor expansion and of the ligaments of the joint with loss of extension. The thumb then falls into the palm at this point, possibly as well as at the carpometacarpal joint, and there may be hyperextension at the interphalangeal joint; both these may become fixed in deformity.

The interphalangeal joint may collapse laterally, usually because of synovitis of the interphalangeal joint and changes away from pad-to-pad opposition.

The digital joints should now be examined starting with the metacarpophalangeal joints.

Metacarpophalangeal joints

These joints are of prime importance in the fingers and often swell from synovial proliferation. As the synovial swelling is surrounded dorsally by the extensor expansion and laterally by the collateral ligaments, both these structures are apt to stretch. As the extensor expansion is usually weaker to the radial side (**Figure 3.15**), stretching is more likely to occur here and, as a result, the extensor tendon is displaced ulnarwards

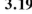

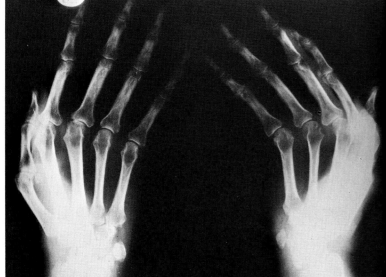

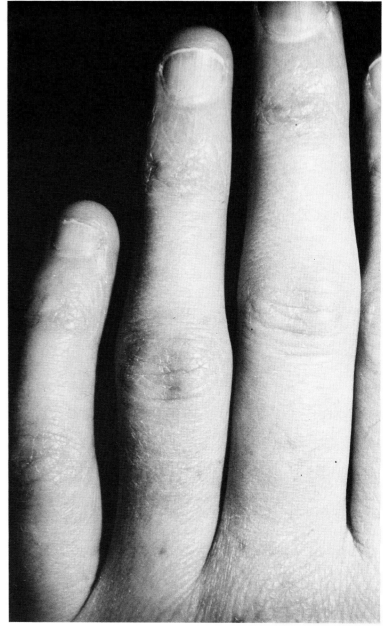

where it slips into the intermetacarpal gutter between the metacarpal heads (**Figure 3.16**). In this position the tendon produces an ulnar deviating force on the digit but loses its effect as a metacarpophalangeal extensor. If the adjacent fingers are held in extension, while the affected finger extends and flexes (**Figure 3.17**) the extensor tendon will pull the radial intrinsic tendon onto the head of the proximal phalanx, where it will prevent flexion of the proximal interphalangeal joint. The sudden release of the intrinsic tendon from this position occurs with an audible and visible snap; this phenomenon is called the 'intrinsic snap' (Harrison 1976).

Proliferating synovial tissues beneath the collateral ligaments erode the underlying bone, the site of the major erosions around the joint, and weaken the attachments and stretch the collateral ligaments, particularly those on the radial side. This allows the digit to drift ulnarwards and – even more important – into volar subluxation. This can be identified on the radiograph using the ball holding view (**Figure 3.18**). Medial shift of the base of the phalanx on the metacarpal head can then be clearly identified. Progressive subluxation leads to limited extension and an established deformity. Ulnar drift can be classified as follows (Harrison 1979):

Grade 1. Dislocation of the extensor tendon without medial shift.
Grade 2. Ulnar drift with medial shift.
Grade 3. Subluxation with ulnar drift and medial shift.
Grade 4. Subluxation, ulnar drift and medial shift with limited passive extension.

Proximal interphalangeal joints

Synovial proliferation causes swelling which can affect, most obviously, the proximal synovial pouch on the dorsum beneath the three slips of the extensor expansion. It can erode the insertion and stretch the central slip (i.e. the extensor of the joint) and it can extend laterally and may bulge through between the central and lateral slips (**Figure 3.19**). It can extend in the joint anteriorly in relation to the volar plate; also, by

affecting the vinculi and bulging of the volar plate it can seriously affect the flexor tendons.

Three deformities can occur at this joint and should be observed:
1   Swan's-neck deformity.
2   Boutonnière.
3   Lateral instability.

Swan's-neck deformity may result from subluxation at the metacarpophalangeal joints; from the intrinsic displacement previously described in the 'intrinsic snap'; it can follow weakening of the proximal attachment of the volar plate, allowing forward displacement, and it can result from intra-articular joint destruction.

It should be recorded if:
1   Voluntary correction is possible.
2   Manual correction is needed.
3   It is not correctable.

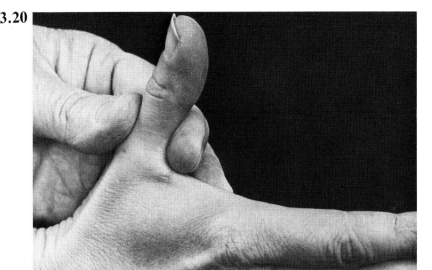

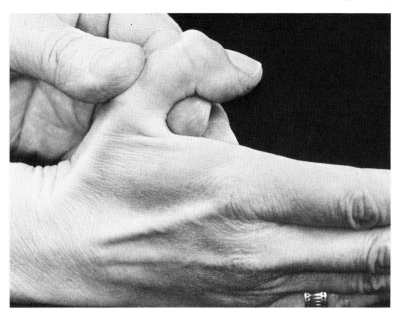

Boutonnière deformity presents in two phases.

1. Complete boutonnière deformity due to disruption of the extensor tendon, in which the joint is flexed to 90° and there is compensatory hyperextension of the terminal joint.

2. Partial boutonnière in which the joint has a flexion deformity of 30–40° with only a moderate degree of hyperextension of the terminal joint.

Lateral instability is seen more often in juvenile rheumatoid arthritis than in adults. The joint is flail and there is little or no function.

Terminal interphalangeal joints

This joint is unusually affected in rheumatoid arthritis (except in the thumb). It is, however, often affected in psoriatic arthritis and in osteoarthrosis.

In psoriatic arthritis, synovitis may be followed by severe joint destruction which may end with a completely flail joint; often, however, the joint may become fused in an abnormal and often afunctional position.

In degenerative or osteoarthrosis new bone commonly forms on the dorsum and presents as nodules called Heberden's nodes. Joint destruction occurs and may be associated with new bone formation. Any limitation of movement and deformity should be recorded.

Degenerative cysts can appear on the dorsum of the joint, owing to extrusion of synovial tissue. The skin may become attenuated and a glairy fluid may be discharged.

Dorsum of the hand

The tendons should now be examined on the dorsum, where synovial swelling around them is commonly seen. This swelling may be associated with rupture of the tendons. As the region of tenosynovium affected is at the wrist it is often difficult to be certain whether the swelling is due to wrist and mid-carpal synovitis or to tenosynovitis. If the wrist is held fixed while the fingers are flexed and extended, movement of the distal end of the swelling with the fingers indicates tenosynovitis. Individual movement of the wrist and each of the digits should then be performed to isolate each tendon as far as possible. Any limitation of movement should be recorded, as this may indicate blocking of tendon movement through the retinaculum, fixation of the tendon because of fibrosing synovitis, or stretching or rupture of a tendon.

When examining the individual tendons it is important to realize that in the prone hand the extensor carpi ulnaris will be running along the ulnar border of the wrist and not over the dorsum.

When the individual tendons are moved actively it is important to record any evidence of pain over the tendon. Pain is often a feature of the period before the tendon ruptures.

A common tendon to rupture is the long extensor of the thumb. This can easily be missed unless examined carefully with the thumb held fully extended (**Figure 3.20**); the patient is then asked to flex and extend his thumb at the interphalangeal joint (**Figure 3.21**). If this method is not used, extension can be camouflaged by the action of the short muscles, particularly the adductor brevis, which can extend the thumb at the interphalangeal joint if some proximal flexion is allowed. The intact extensor pollicis longus will usually stand out when the thumb is extended (**Figure 3.22**) but this may not be obvious when there is severe tenosynovitis.

The other common extensor tendon rupture is to the little finger, followed by that to the ring finger. There is failure to extend the finger at the metacarpophalangeal joint (interphalangeal extension can be brought about by the intrinsic muscles). However, a similar effect can be seen after dislocation of the extensor tendons off the metacarpal head into the intermetacarpal gutter or after a severe volar subluxation at the metacarpophalangeal joint. If the tendon is ruptured there will be no sign of the tendon standing out over the dorsum of the metacarpal when extension is attempted (**Figure 3.23**).

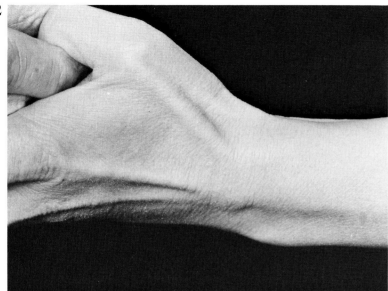

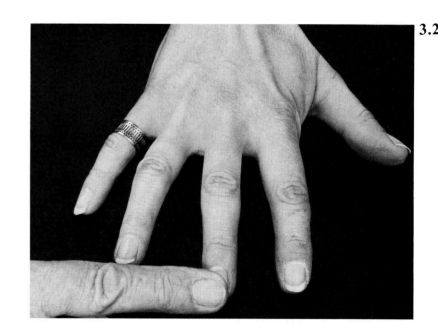

Palmar aspect of the hand

Synovial swelling around the tendons on the palmar aspect of the hand must be considered in two parts. The proximal palmar bursa extends from proximal to the wrist crease to approximately the level of the proximal transverse palmar crease. The digital synovial sheaths then begin at about the distal palmar crease and extend into the digit to the insertion of the tendons. The thumb flexor has its own separate sheath extending through its length and in the case of the little finger there may be continuity from the palmar bursa into the finger. As stated previously, it is not easy to assess the state of tenosynovium affected in the palm without considerable experience, though florid spread is usually readily apparent. Often the presence of the thickened synovium can be surmised by evidence of carpal-tunnel compression of the median nerve as shown by paraesthesia (mainly nocturnal) in the median-nerve sensory area, or weakness of the thenar muscles. Direct pressure on the nerve or acute flexion of the wrist may both initiate paraesthesia in carpal-tunnel compression.

When considering loss of thenar muscle bulk it is important to remember that this occurs quite commonly, as does loss of interosseous power and bulk, as a result of disuse atrophy in rheumatoid and other arthropathies and therefore must be differentiated from that due to a nerve lesion.

Palpation over the flexor tendons as the fingers are flexed either actively or passively may give evidence of synovial bulk. This may be found proximal to the carpal tunnel by palpating the tendons medial to palmaris longus (i.e. the flexor digitorum superficialis or sublimis tendons) (**Figure 3.24**). Also, with the fingers in the same position, pressure in the centre of the palm may force fluid proximally if there is much synovial fluid; occasionally, tapping in the palm may produce a 'thrill'.

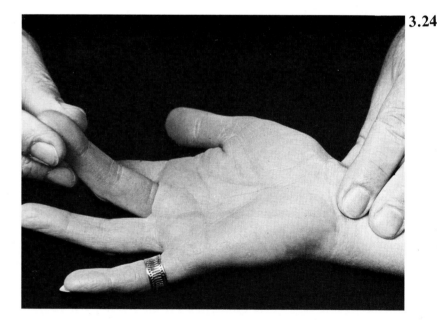

3.25

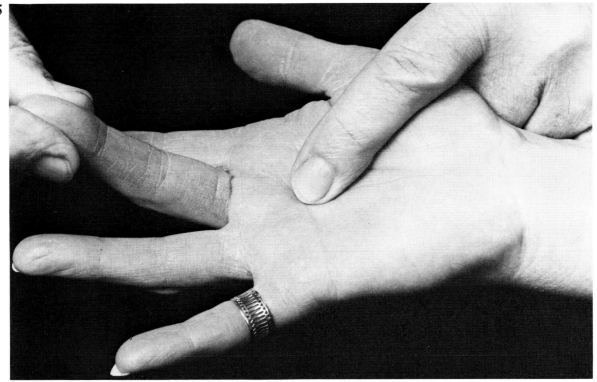

3.26

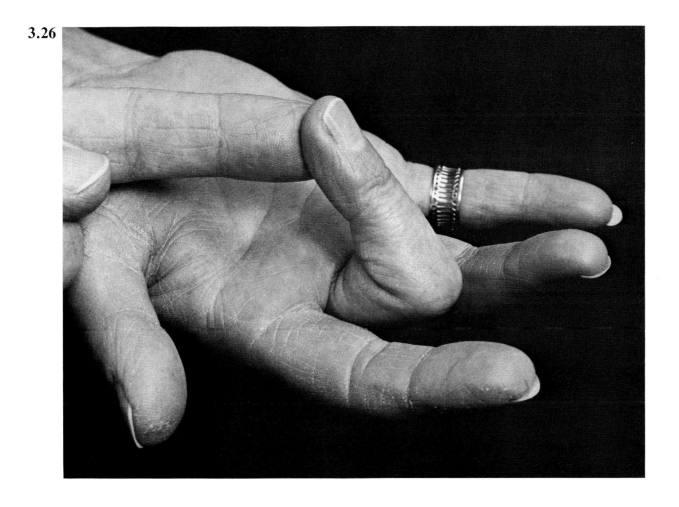

3.27

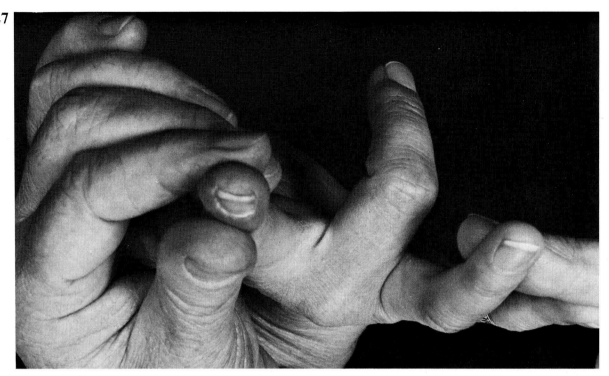

Only if there is a great deal of synovial bulk associated with softening of the flexor retinaculum, as often does occur, will evidence of bulk be palpable beneath the ligament but it is usually palpable on digital flexion and extension in the interval between the distal end of the retinaculum and the palmar bursa, i.e. between the level of the outstretched thumb and the proximal palmar crease.

Triggering of the finger is commonly evidence of digital disease. There may be some bulging in the region of the distal palmar crease with the finger extended. Palpation over this point as the finger is passively flexed and extended (**Figure 3.25**) will indicate the build up of retained bulk of synovium as the finger is extended, or evidence of the bulk being squeezed into the digital fibrous flexor sheath.

Pressure over the synovial bulk may give pain. This sometimes indicates quite severe tendon damage.

The close bunching of the flexor tendons in the palmar synovial bursa often leads to severe tendon damage and sometimes rupture. The tendons may become matted together, as a mass of surrounding synovial tissue, contained granulomata and necrotic tendon, thus producing a mass action.

Evidence of this may be produced by testing the separate activities of the two long flexor muscles. Flexor digitorum profundus can be tested by hooking the fingers at the terminal phalanx. Flexor digitorum superficialis (sublimis) is less easy. The finger can be flexed at the proximal interphalangeal joint, keeping the distal joint extended (**Figure 3.26**) or each finger can be flexed in turn whilst the examiner holds the remainder in extension, thus isolating the superficial flexor (**Figure 3.27**).

If the actions cannot be separated there may be a conjoined palmar mass and on occasions one or other tendon may even be ruptured in the palm but retain some continuity through the synovial material.

Flexor tendon rupture can occur in the palm, usually at the distal end of the retinaculum, but more commonly affects the long flexor of the thumb than the fingers.

Flexor pollicis longus may rupture in one of three places:

1   In the thenar compartment.
2   At the level of the metacarpophalangeal joint.
3   Avulsion from its distal attachment.

Rupture of the long flexor tendon is recognized by holding the thumb fully extended and asking the patient to flex and extend the terminal joint as for the extensor tendon (**Figure 3.20** and **3.21**).

3.28

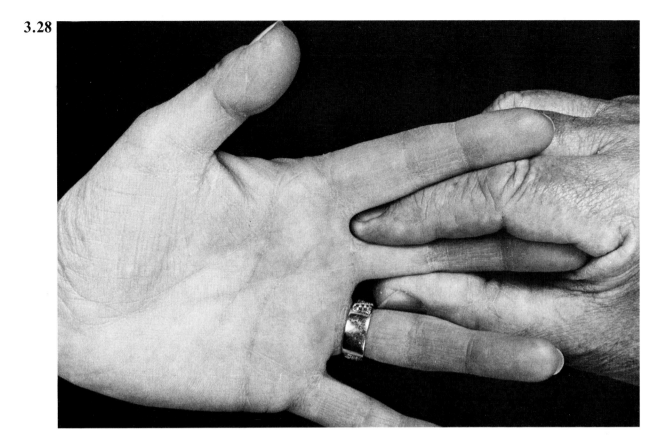

Within the digits

Proliferation of the flexor synovial sheath may be identified by lateral compression at the level of the proximal phalanx (**Figure 3.28**). If there is much thickening of synovium, the skin will not crease on the surface and it will not be possible to approximate the skin on pressure. At the same time a bulging of soft tissue may be seen.

Often the flexor tendons may be affected in relation to the proximal interphalangeal joints, either because of bulging of the volar plate from within the joint or because of the vincular synovium being affected, or both.

Palpation over the region as the finger is flexed may indicate such a problem.

It is often useful to prepare a proforma so that the examination can be systematized. In all cases there should be photographs of the hands, radiographs taken in at least three views, and measurements recorded on a die stamp of flexor and extensor deficit of the fingers or other abnormalities, as previously stated.

4: Nerve and tenosynovial compressions and other conditions

To control tendons without producing bow-stringing, the wrist and hand are equipped with a number of retinaculi; these are found on the flexor and extensor aspects at the wrist and the fibrous flexor sheaths of the fingers. To these may be added several fibrous arcades beneath which nerves pass. Pathology of various types at these sites commonly needs surgical intervention. Compressions can occur to the median nerve as it passes behind a possible supracondylar spur, or beneath the origins of pronator teres or flexor digitorum sublimis (superficialis), or, in particular, in the carpal tunnel; to the ulnar nerve in the cubital tunnel behind the medial humeral epicondyle or beneath the superficial slip of the flexor retinaculum; and to the posterior interosseous nerve as it passes through supinator onto the dorsum of the arm. Tight fibro-osseous tunnels or tenosynovial thickening can also limit the easy movement of tendons beneath retinaculi, producing tenosynovial stress and thus further synovial inflammatory bulk. These conditions require either a release of the compressing fibrous bands, though obviously without loss of retinacular control, or removal of the limiting synovial bulk, or both.

Median nerve

A supracondylar spur occasionally leads to compression of the nerve which runs with the artery behind the spur and then passes forwards beneath the ligament linking the spur with the medial epicondyle. The nerve, if compressed, should be transposed anteriorly by dividing the ligament at the spur. If the ulnar head of pronator teres has a high origin from the ligament, it should be repaired after transposition of the nerve. Occasionally the median nerve may be compressed by fibrous arches as it passes beneath pronator teres or flexor digitorum sublimis (superficialis). This can be relieved by simple division of the constricting bands, care being taken not to divide too much of the overlying muscle.

The most common site of median nerve compression is the carpal tunnel.

Carpal-tunnel syndrome

Although this condition is fairly common, it is often not treated until it has become quite severe, and severe sensory or motor loss has occurred. In such cases the chances of recovery after appropriate treatment are uncertain. Presentation is five times more common in women than in men, and more common in the older age group, i.e. the menopausal or postmenopausal years. In younger women it is sometimes a feature of pregnancy, or symptoms may appear or become worse in the premenstrual period of fluid retention. In males, as in females, it tends to be a condition of older age groups; but in both sexes cases are not uncommon in younger people, particularly after trauma.

Characteristically, the patient wakes at night with paraesthesiae and often pain in the median nerve distribution in the hand. The same symptoms may be present by day but are almost always worse at night due to fluid retention during sleep. Very commonly the patient complains of pain running proximally up the arm to the elbow and even to the axilla or shoulder. Thus a high proportion of cases of carpal-tunnel syndrome are missed as the clinician's thoughts are directed to a lesion of the cervical spine such as osteoarthrosis, a disc prolapse, the much publicized but quite rare thoracic-inlet syndrome, or a cervical rib. Sometimes there may be complaints of frank numbness or weakness of the fingers.

Physical examination may often be relatively inconclusive in early cases, but an early diagnosis is important in any nerve compression if permanent disability is to be limited.

Observation may detect very little. Reduced sensibility may be found, whether touch, pin-prick or two-point discrimination. There may be weakness of thumb opposition and abduction and in late cases a frank hollowing of the thenar eminence owing to loss of the abductor, part of flexor pollicis brevis and the underlying opponens muscles.

Paraesthesia in the fingers may be elicited by a Tinel test – i.e. tapping the wrist over the median nerve – or more reliably by sustained thumb pressure for 30–60 seconds over the nerve at the wrist – i.e. between the flexor carpi radialis and palmaris longus tendons. Full extension or flexion at the wrist for a similar period may also induce paraesthesiae, as may inflation of a sphygmomanometer cuff to midway between the arterial and venous pressures, so increasing fluid pressure in the limb. Perhaps the most sensitive test is measurement by electromyography of a motor conduction time or, more reliably, of the sensory conduction time of the median nerve across the carpal tunnel. The enthusiast for clinical measurement will often say that this last technique is the only reliable test but even here discrepancies arise. Owing to the wide variation in normal conduction time across the wrist (3–5 milliseconds) the normal rate of a patient with a normally fast conduction time could well have almost doubled and still be within the general normal limit. It is therefore important to compare the worst (usually the dominant) hand with the less affected. In many cases there may be a normal basic conduction time but a secondary conduction peak a little later indicates a conduction delay in some of the nerve fibres. In severe cases there may be electromyographic evidence of positive or total denervation in the thenar muscles. The diagnosis of the more proximal compressions of the median nerve is usually made after excluding the possibility of a carpal-tunnel compression. In these cases, the nocturnal symptoms are usually less severe, as the tenosynovium is unaffected. Nerve conduction times over segments of the nerve accurately indicate the region of compression. A supracondylar conduction delay can be confirmed radiologically by showing the presence of a supracondylar spur.

Carpal-tunnel compression can often be treated conservatively, especially if it is short-standing, but if there is much delay in the normal conduction time or significant clinical sensory or motor loss has occurred, surgical decompression will probably be necessary. An effective division of the carpal ligament is essential, avoiding damage to the palmar cutaneous branch of the median nerve or the thenar motor branch which, contrary to the usual anatomical descriptions, usually arises from the volar aspect of the nerve trunk in the tunnel, where it can be extremely vulnerable. Incisions should be limited as much as possible, but quite often it is advisable to carry out a tenosynovectomy at the same time if there is marked synovial thickening (nearly all carpal-tunnel compressions are associated with thickened tenosynovium). A selection of incisions is shown on **Figure 4.1**.

If a short incision is to be used, giving a relatively blind approach to the carpal ligament, incision A in the thenar crease has the advantage of preserving the palmar branch of the median nerve and allowing the operator to see the branches,

particularly the thenar branch, in the palm. If there is any need for full opening of the region – for example, to expose the tendons for a synovectomy – the incision can easily be extended proximally. Incision B allows a direct approach to the ligament but leaves a scar over the heel of the hand. Damage to the palmar nerve or its branches may cause postoperative pain and tenderness in a very unacceptable part of the hand. Incision C leaves a highly acceptable scar but the palmar cutaneous branch must be approached very carefully; a postoperative neuroma at the heel of the hand is a very severe disability. Incision D runs across crease lines and sometimes thickens and, as with incision C, the operator has no means of knowing whether the thenar motor branch is intact. It is often difficult to know how far distally to pass the knife; if the superficial palmar arch is cut or the knife slips between the laminae, bypassing the distal deeper fibres of the retinaculum, the patient is often left without relief.

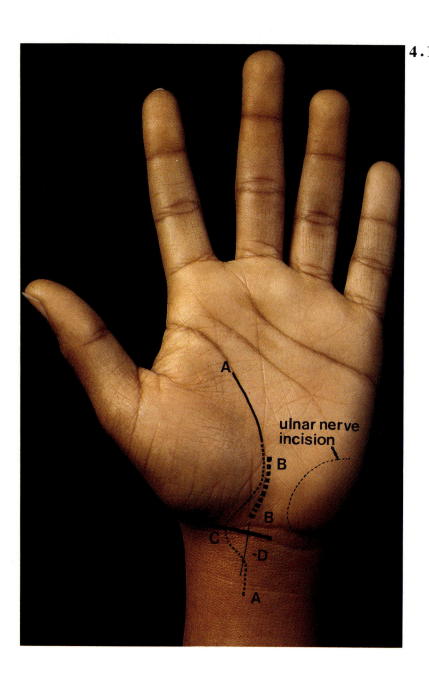

4.1

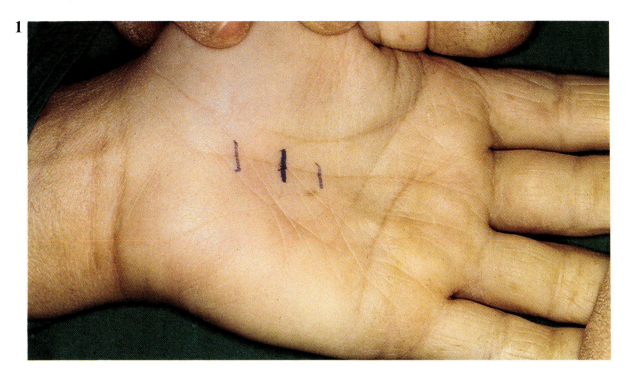

Simple carpal-tunnel decompression

1 A common incision is in the thenar crease but if, as in this case, there is a second crease more ulnarwards this is to be preferred, so lessening the risk of damage to the thenar, motor branch of the median nerve.

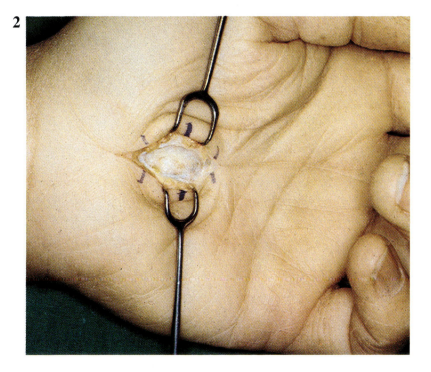

2 The incision is made carefully through the distal part of the flexor retinaculum and the palmar aponeurosis, avoiding cutting the syperficial palmar vascular arch. It is now possible to ascertain the position of the median nerve in the palm.

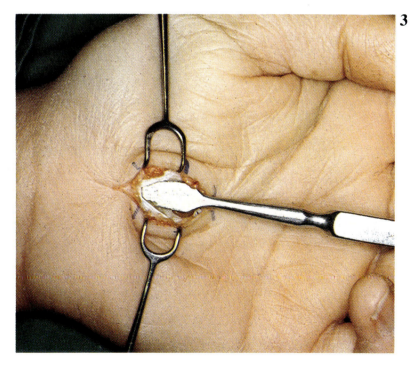

3 A guide is passed, keeping to the ulnar side of the median nerve. The guide must not be forced even in a tight tunnel, for it can easily damage an early branch of the median nerve, particularly the thenar motor branch in the carpal tunnel. If the guide cannot be passed easily, a blind approach should be abandoned and the incision extended proximally to give an open approach.

4

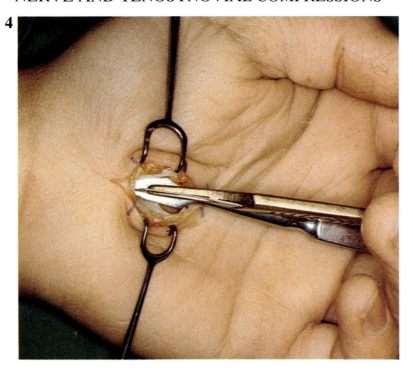

5

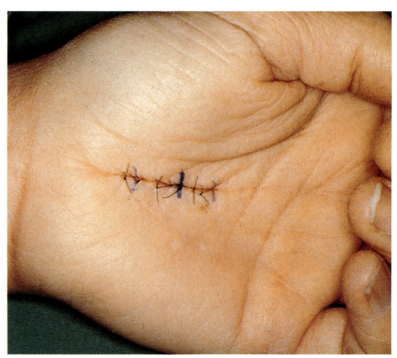

4 A narrow-bladed knife can now be slipped in with its back to the guide until the retinaculum can be felt to give way throughout its length. The incision should be directed just to the ulnar side of palmaris longus (if present) so as to avoid damage to the palmar branch of the median nerve. Care must also be taken to limit the division to the retinacular fibres so as to avoid damage to the more superficial palmar branch of the median nerve.

5 The wound can now be sutured. It is advisable to warn the patient that the scar might be a little hypersensitive for a few months postoperatively but will then become painless.

Ulnar nerve

Compressions here are usually identified by paraesthesiae or reduced sensibility in the ulnar nerve innervated fingers and sometimes weakness or loss of bulk in the muscles supplied by the nerve. A positive Tinel test at the elbow or wrist may indicate the site, which can then be confirmed by nerve conduction tests.

The ulnar nerve is particularly vulnerable in the cubital tunnel, where it lies subcutaneously behind the medial epicondyle of the humerus. Here it is vulnerable to external trauma or compression beneath the fibrous arch formed by the origins of flexor carpi ulnaris over the epicondyle. Pathology of either the epicondyle or its covering can reduce the diameter of the tunnel, or thickening of the nerve from any cause can produce a self-aggravating compression. Increase of the carrying angle after supracondylar fractures for instance, can lead to stretching of the nerve through the fixed tunnel.

Traditionally, compression at the elbow has been treated by anterior transposition of the nerve, but this requires wide exposure and freeing of the nerve, possibly damaging nerve branches close to the elbow and occasionally causing secondary compression from other anatomical structures. Transposition is still to be recommended if there is proven tightness in length, but in most cases a simple division of the covering fibres is all that is required. Osborn (1970) recommends placing the divided fibres beneath the nerve but this often means loss of the branch to the elbow joint. In our experience simple division and local excision of the roof of the tunnel is usually all that is

required. The operation is thus reduced from a fairly major to a minor procedure.

Occasionally an ulnar nerve is not effectively constrained in the cubital tunnel and is free to flick around the medial epicondyle. This may give little more than periodic discomfort, but sometimes when the nerve becomes vulnerable to damage it is worth attempting to construct a cubital bridge or, since the nerve is already free to move around the epicondyle, to complete its anterior freedom by a surgical anterior transposition.

At the wrist the ulnar nerve passes beneath the superficial slip of the carpal ligament and alongside the pisiform bone, where it divides into its superficial and deep branches. Compression in the tunnel of either of the divisions can occur. The site can normally be determined clinically, permitting an accurate approach to the region of compression.

The nerve can be approached by lifting a flap which includes the palmaris brevis muscle. The main nerve trunk and then the branches can be traced and any constricting band or swelling can be removed. It is advisable to try to preserve the palmaris brevis muscle, including its nerve supply, for by bunching the soft tissues over the ulnar nerve this muscle provides considerable protection from external trauma.

Compressions of the posterior interosseous nerve are uncommon other than after trauma or a fractured radius, but they should be considered when there is otherwise unexplained weakness in the muscles on the posterior aspect of the forearm.

Tenosynovial compression

This can occur at any site where a tendon passes under a fibrous arch which for some reason becomes too tight. In some cases the fibrous binding and constrictions may be secondary to trauma or other post-inflammatory fibrosis. Where they occur in relation to usually positioned anatomical fibrous arches the tendon will have a synovial sheath which will also play a major part in the eventual pathology. The most common sites for such compressions are the entrance to the fibrous flexor sheath of the finger producing 'trigger finger', with a comparable condition in the thumb, and the point at which the abductor

pollicis longus and extensor pollicis brevis tendons pass under the extensor retinaculum – De Quervain's syndrome. These conditions are often called tenovaginitis stenosans or stenosing tendovaginitis, indicating that the primary condition is a stenosis or tightening of the fibrous arch or a fibrosis of the synovium. While such fibrous constrictions do often occur, the primary cause is more commonly thickened inflammatory synovitis due to trauma or non-specific or rheumatoid disease; the fibrous sheath then becomes constrictive on the thick tenosynovium. Quite often a patient presenting for the first time with strong evidence of rheumatoid disease will have had treatment for a trigger finger, De Quervain's syndrome or a carpal-tunnel compression in preceding months.

Ulnar nerve decompression

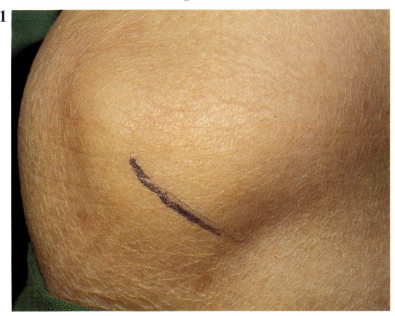

1 The elbow is prepared and a suture relocation mark made across the ulnar nerve.

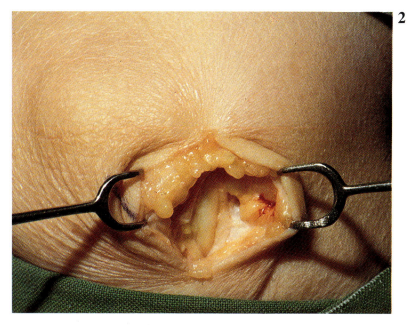

3 The aponeurosis is opened from the proximal edge and extended distally until the compression region has been cleared.

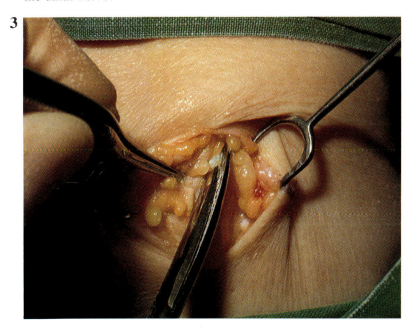

2 A short incision is made from just proximal to the medial epicondyle along the line of the ulnar nerve. The aponeurosis can be seen over the nerve.

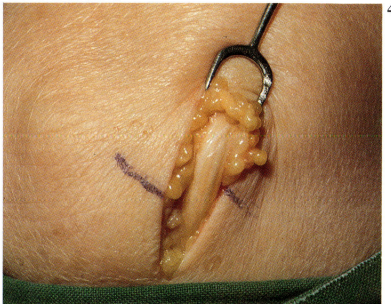

4 The nerve is now lying free, showing some thinning where the fibres originally arched over.

Trigger finger

Trigger finger. The initial symptom is usually difficulty in extending the finger after it has been flexed into the palm. The condition is usually worse in the morning until the fluid retention of sleep has dispersed. The patient often has to use the other hand to initiate extension because of the mechanical disadvantage of the extensors at full flexion, or the finger may be extended initially with difficulty, flicking out with the so-called 'trigger' effect. There may be simple disproportion between the fibrous flexor sheath and tendon but more commonly there is severe tenosynovitis. The tenosynovial bulk is pulled out of the fibrous sheath on flexion and then has to be forced back in again. Because of the tightness of the sheath, a thickened mass is held in the palm as the finger extends. This stress on the synovium aggravates the inflammatory state. The mass of synovium is usually to be felt in the region of the distal flexor crease in the palm when the finger is flexed and its movement is obvious as the finger is extended. There may be pain in this region on extension of the finger; there may even be pain in the region of the proximal interphalangeal joint, probably because of stress on the extensor system. The synovial bulk also gives pain on pressure.

Some mild synovitic cases can be effectively treated by rest and hydrocortisone and local anaesthetic injection. Many however, will require surgical intervention. A short incision along the distal flexor crease will reveal the thickened synovium, the proximal end of the digital synovial sheath and the proximal free margin of the fibrous flexor sheath. In many cases a simple local synovectomy of the tendons, pulling them as far into the palm with the finger flexed as much as possible, is all that is required. If, however, the fibrous flexor sheath appears too tight and thickened, the proximal centimetre or so may be excised. It is important not to excise too much of the fibrous flexor sheath or the tendon will bow-string on flexion and limit the range of digital flexion.

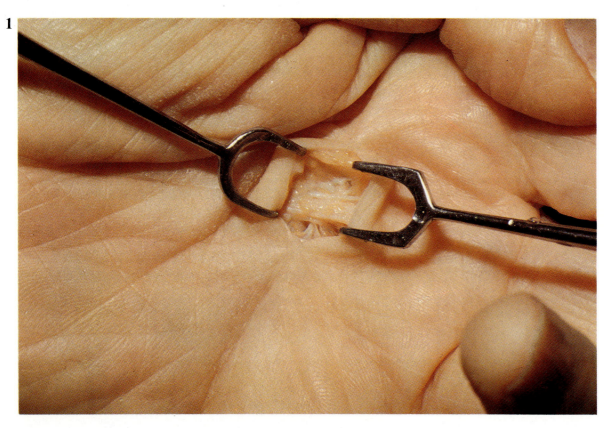

1 A small incision is made in the distal flexor crease over the offending tendon. It need only be long enough to admit a pair of double hook retractors (or cat's-paws).

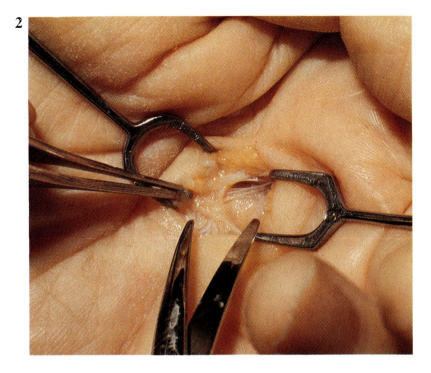

2 The palmar aponeurosis is divided longitudinally to expose the underlying tendons.

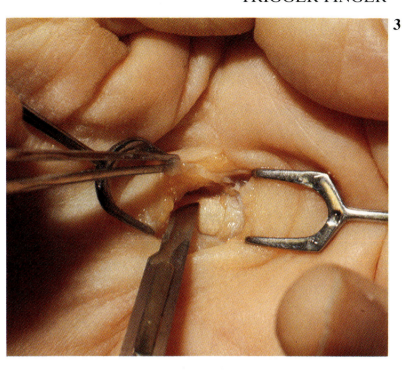

3 The tenosynovium can now be removed, first on the superficialis (sublimis) and then on the deeper profundus tendon. This will be facilitated by pulling out the tendons with blunt hooks, flexing the fingers to the maximum into the palm. Thus much digital length of tendon can be cleaned.

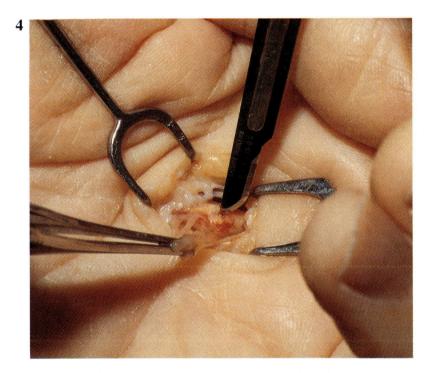

4 If the fibrous flexor sheath is too tight for the tendons at its proximal end it can be divided, or a short piece (up to 1 cm in length) can be removed to allow free movement.

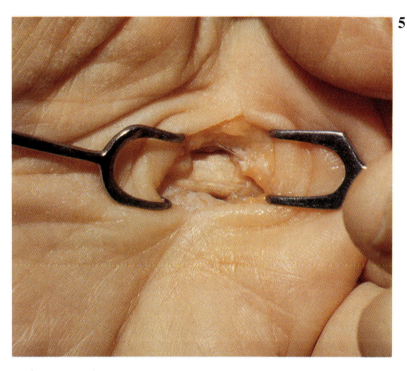

5 This division need rarely be more than a few millimetres, leaving a satisfactory sling over the proximal digital phalanx.

Trigger thumb

Trigger thumb. This is a similar condition to trigger finger but occurs at the volar aspect of the metacarpophalangeal joint. A thickened synovial nodule is often present on the flexor pollicis longus tendon. An incision along the flexor crease of the joint gives adequate exposure for the removal of the offending synovium. It is essential when using this incision to remember that the digital nerves in the thumb can be remarkably variable in their course at this point, and great care must be taken not to damage either the main nerve or a major branch running on the volar aspect of the joint.

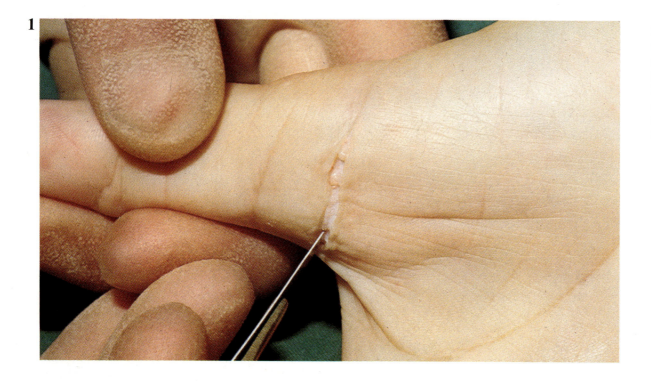

1 The incision is made along the metacarpophalangeal flexor crease. The sensory nerve of the radial border of the thumb is likely to be crossing the volar aspect immediately beneath the skin of the incision line and hence is highly vulnerable.

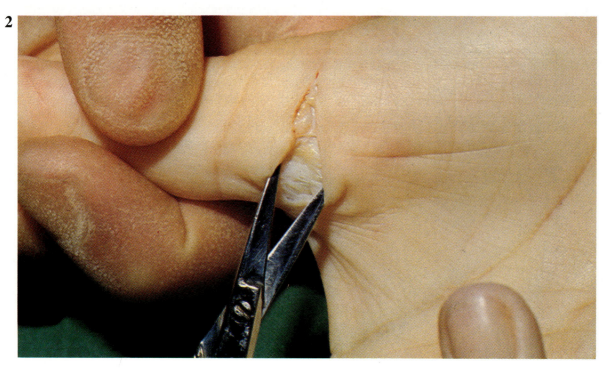

2 If the incision is carefully limited to the skin, the edges can be separated by blunt dissection and nerves and vessels isolated as they cross the field. The digital nerve can be seen beside the points of the scissors.

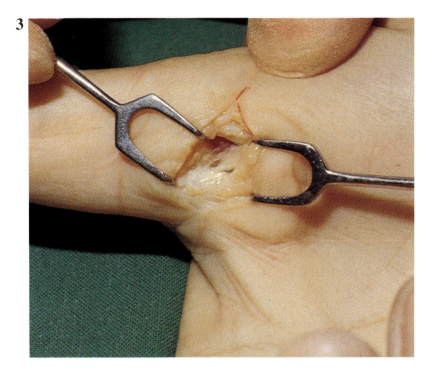

3 The nerve and any vessel can be pushed laterally by the double skin hooks which are also retracting the skin. The fibrous flexor sheath is now exposed.

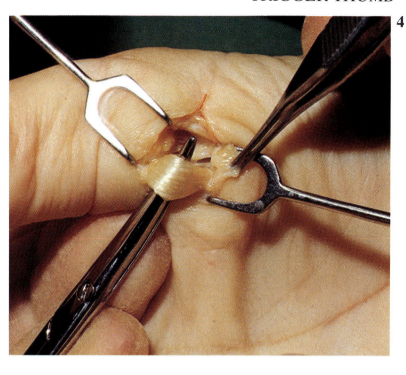

4 The sheath is divided to expose the tendon and the constricting band or synovial swelling is isolated and removed.

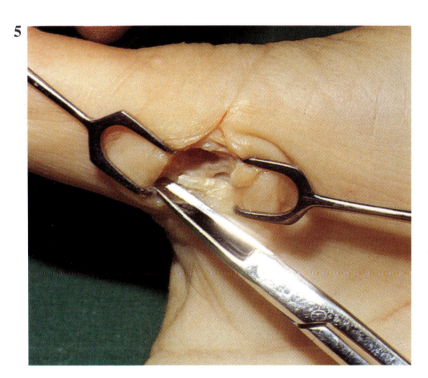

5 The fibrous flexor sheath can be divided and removed for a few millimetres up the thumb to clear the constricted area.

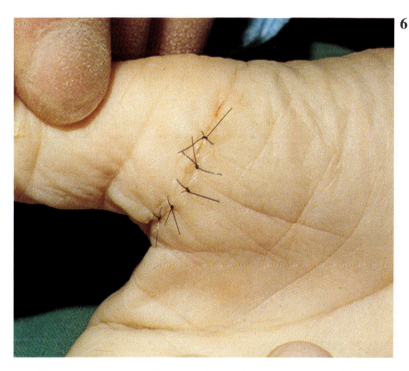

6 The wound is sutured. Being in the flexor crease no visible scar will be expected.

De Quervain

De Quervain's syndrome. This is characterized by pain proximal to the radial styloid on gripping or movement at the wrist, particularly that giving radial deviation. Sometimes the condition begins after unaccustomed exercise, usually in a woman, but there may be no obvious cause. Onset may be a gradual swelling over the tendons of abductor pollicis longus and extensor pollicis brevis. Pain on exercise may radiate up the arm or into the thumb. If the hand is passively carried into ulnar deviation, pain is elicited in the region of the radial styloid; this can be quite severe so the test should be made gently.

The condition can be treated by rest in full plaster (not a volar slab, as this allows muscle activity), hydrocortisone and local anaesthetic injection, or by injection alone. Despite this quite severe conservative regimen the recurrence rate is high and surgical decompression then becomes necessary. For this reason, except in mild cases or cases of recent onset, it is common to advise surgery and so avoid a long, incapacitated wait for a possible improvement.

The incision varies with the surgeon. Many prefer a wide exposure and use a longitudinal incision in the line of the tendons. This has the advantage that there is less risk of damaging the radial nerve branches. However, the incision crosses crease and stress lines and may sometimes leave a less acceptable scar in a very obvious place, particularly in a woman who may wish to wear short sleeves. To avoid this the longitudinal incision is sometimes converted to a Z-plastic. A transverse incision gives adequate exposure, remembering that the skin in this area is mobile; this incision leaves an inconspicuous scar. The disadvantage of the transverse incision, despite the ease of access, is that it crosses important radial nerve branches which must be isolated and retained, thus complicating the exposure. Nevertheless it is usually the incision of choice. The tendons of abductor pollicis longus and extensor pollicis brevis will be found beneath their retinaculum, which must be divided longitudinally to expose the tendons and their synovial sheath. Opening the fibro-osseous compartment is often considered sufficient, but this limited tenosynovial freeing may result in continued though reduced disability. As the synovial membrane is usually thickened either as a primary or secondary pathology it is advisable to carry out a local synovectomy of the tendons. This can be done quite easily by mobilizing the hand and the tendon about the incision so that a considerable synovial length can be removed, even through the small transverse incision.

It is important to free the complete length of both muscle tendons beneath the retinaculum. There is considerable variation in these tendons and their coverings; for example abductor pollicis longus usually has two tendons and may have three or more at this region, and extensor pollicis brevis may only be a thin tendon or may even be absent. These variations are not always appreciated and clearance may be incomplete as a result.

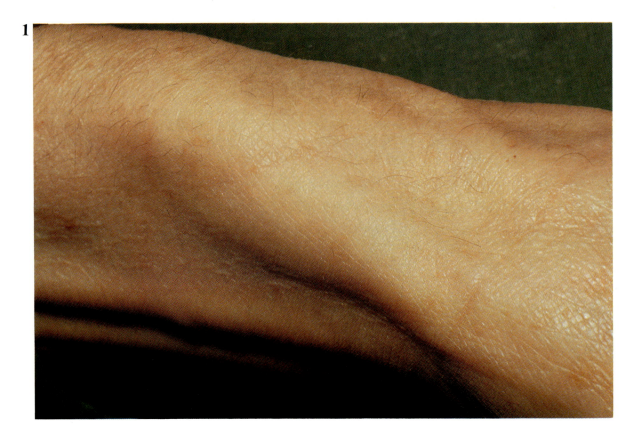

1 The thickened tenosynovium can be seen beneath the skin. A longitudinal incision is often used giving a better exposure with less chance of nerve damage. However, an incision in a crease line gives a far better scar and, with care, is safe and gives adequate exposure.

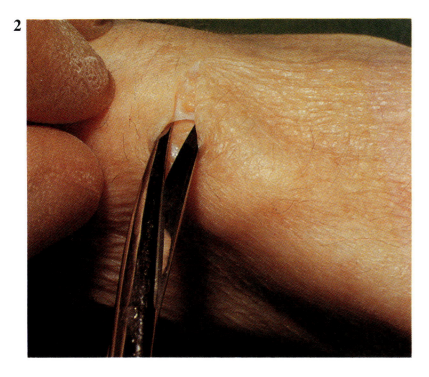

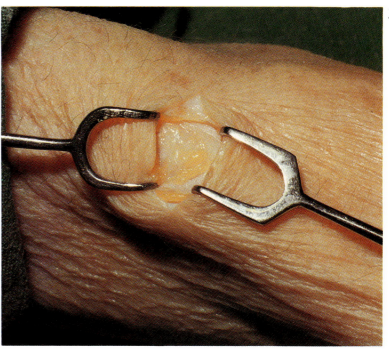

2 A small incision is made towards the proximal end of the retinaculum. The incision should be skin deep, so as to preserve the small nerve branches. If the wound is widened by scissors the branches can be seen and preserved.

3 The nerve branches can be mobilized and double hooks can be used to retract skin between the nerves, giving a nerve-clear area over the affected tendons.

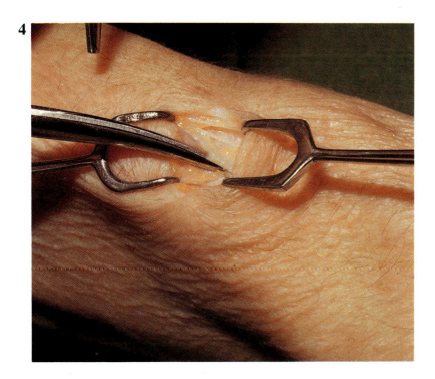

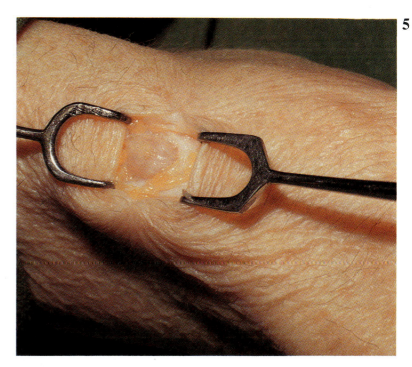

4 A scalpel incision through the retinaculum can be extended proximally and distally by the use of blunt pointed (e.g. MacIndoe) dissecting scissors. At the same time the mobile skin is pulled proximally and distally, giving quite adequate exposure even from the small incision.

5 The thickened, inflamed tenosynovium is thus exposed. Once the retinacular compression has been removed the condition will often settle without further problems.

6

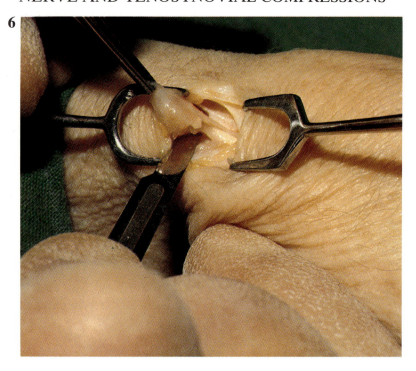

7

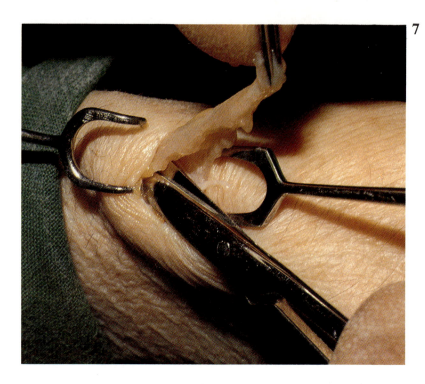

6 As the tenosynovium is exposed it is our practice to remove it. This produces better results.

7 Using the same basic techniques as in dividing the retinaculum, almost the whole length of the tenosynovium can be excised. This is easier if the wrist is moved through its full range to give maximal tendon excursion in relation to the incision.

8

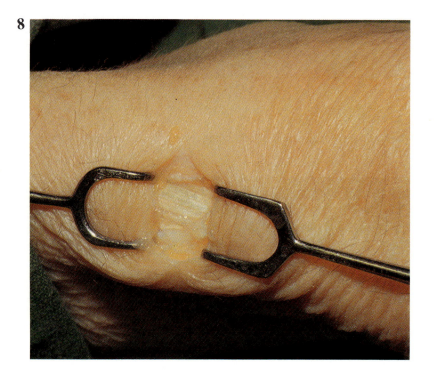

8 The tendon can be left in a clean state to allow more normal tenosynovial regeneration. Sometimes, even in this local condition, surface damage of the tendon can be found. When checking that all the tendons are clear and free, it is important to remember that the abductor pollicis longus usually has more than one tendon.

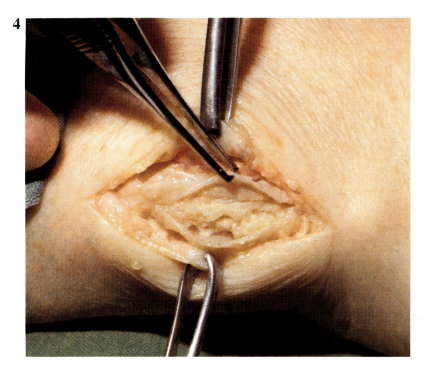

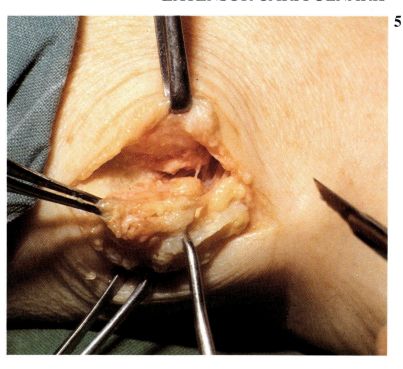

4 Sometimes, as in this case, the core of the tendon may become totally necrotic but this tendon, unlike most others, often retains a thick, fibrous, intact coat. This coat has been opened to expose the necrotic contents.

5 Much of the necrotic core is removed.

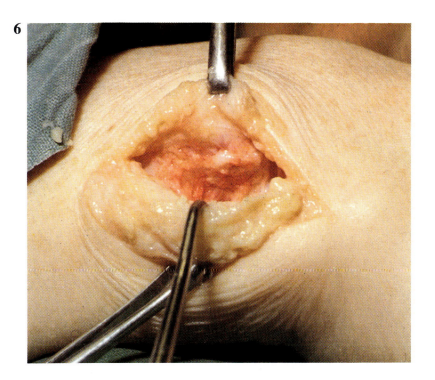

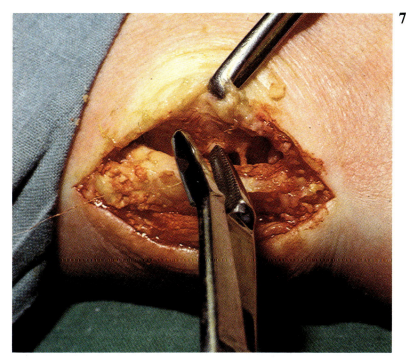

6 The tendon bed is cleared and the erosions in the ulna are thoroughly cleared.

7 The tourniquet has been released and the bleeding controlled. If suction drainage is used postoperatively this is less important; but here bleeding might occur and a drain is impractical. The tendon is repaired using Dexon (or Prolene or similar material).

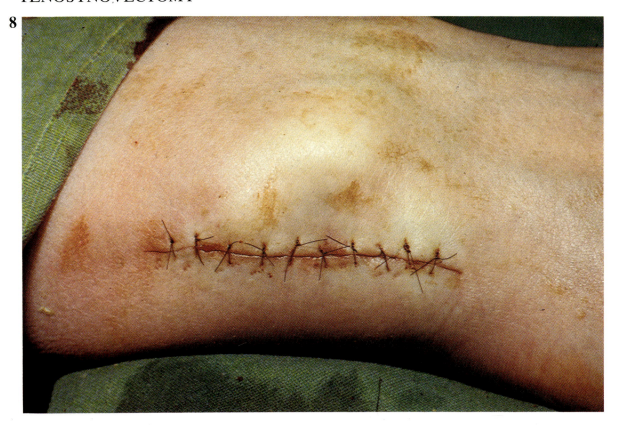

8 The wound is sutured.

Flexor tenosynovectomy

This varies according to the region of the flexor tendons affected. The synovial sheath extends through the palmar bursa, and then through a gap and into the fingers. Thus the main sites for operation are the palmar bursa and the digital sheath at the entrance to the fibrous flexor sheath or within the finger. All of these can be affected to varying degrees and can be treated individually, or occasionally a complete synovectomy may be called for.

A satisfactory incision for the palmar bursa follows the line of the thenar flexor crease with a marked curve across the wrist creases and then up the forearm as far as necessary. The proximal ends of the synovial sheaths of the digital tendons may extend more proximally in rheumatoid disease than in the normal hand, sometimes even as far as the muscle belly.

When making the incision it is important to watch for and preserve the palmar cutaneous branch of the median nerve which normally travels to the medial side of the tendon of flexor carpi radialis. Division of this small nerve can produce severe disturbances if a neuroma forms at the heel of the hand.

If the digital sheaths are only slightly affected the palmar bursa may be severely affected, and vice versa. Often the digital sheath may be affected only near the entrance to the fibrous flexor sheath or more distally. If the sheath is affected more distally, the finger must be opened either laterally or by a zig-zag incision on the volar aspect (e.g. a Bruner incision). On a single finger, particularly the index or middle finger, this can be carried through from the palmar incision.

In many cases there is a large mass at the entrance of the fibrous flexor sheath, which can usually be dealt with quite effectively by an incision along the distal palmar crease to expose the tendons. The synovium can be removed proximally to the fibrous flexor sheath but the tendons must then be pulled out into the palm. This completely flexes the finger and a large mass of synovium, often with disrupted tendon, will be exposed. The tendon may well have normal synovium more distally. It is often said that a distal synovectomy at the entrance to the fingers produces a disproportionate amount of fibrosis. This is certainly true if there is wide exposure and undermining of the skin, but if the operation is kept very local and the tendon is pulled as required, a large area of tendon can be dealt with quite simply. This produces very satisfactory results, including excellent postoperative mobility in most cases.

Further distally in the finger there is the region near the proximal interphalangeal joint, which should also be considered seriously because of the concurrent effects on the joint and the vinculi.

Whatever treatment is carried out on the finger, it is very important to preserve the fibrous flexor sheath bands. These occasionally become stretched after long-standing synovial swelling so that after synovectomy or natural improvement they become too slack to allow full flexion. It may be necessary to tighten up or replace the band over the proximal phalanx to allow recovery of full digital flexion.

Proximal flexor synovectomy

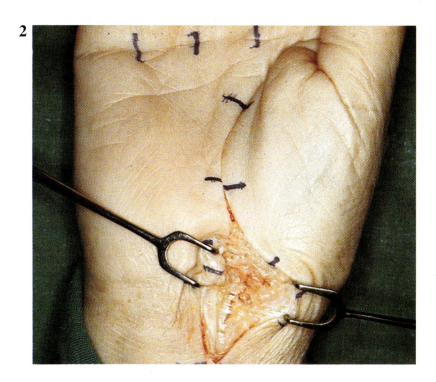

1 This can be carried out using an incision following the thenar crease and across the wrist as shown. In this case, marks have also been made across the distal palmar crease, since there is a distal synovial bulk present.

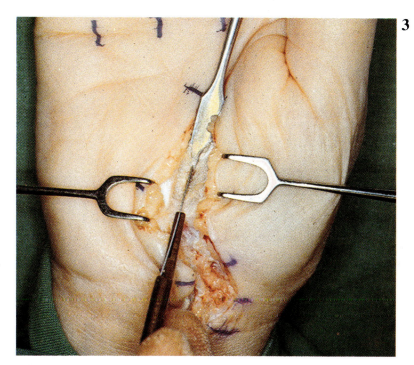

2 The skin is reflected at the heel of the hand to locate the palmar branch of the median nerve before dividing the retinaculum. A neuroma formed after a cut palmar nerve branch at the heel of the hand can be highly painful.

3 The palmar fascia is divided distal to the retinaculum taking care to preserve the superficial palmar arterial arch. It is advisable also to find the thenar branch of the median nerve. A McDonald or similar elevator is passed under the retinaculum, well to the ulnar side, and the retinaculum divided. Care should be taken; the median nerve is often pushed ulnarwards by synovial bulk and the thenar branch may come off from the ulnar side of the main nerve.

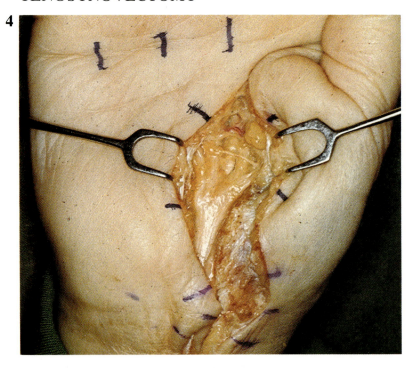

4 Check that the thenar branch is safe after opening the tunnel. In this case it comes off the front of the radial side and passes through the retinaculum into the thenar muscles – a very common variant.

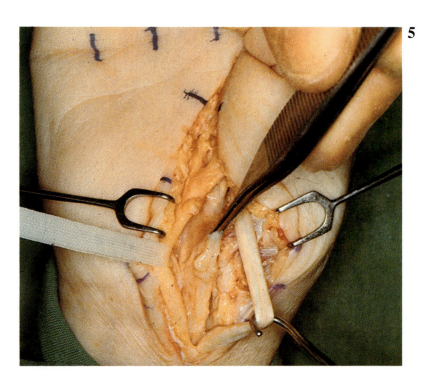

5 The median nerve is dissected from the surrounding tissues. Often it is firmly bound to these tissues and has to be cut free. A tape has been passed round the nerve, which is retracted ulnarwards to allow access to the tendon of flexor pollicis longus. This is commonly lightly covered in the palm and as in this case easily cleaned and pulled out on a hook. The thick synovium can be seen on the other tendons.

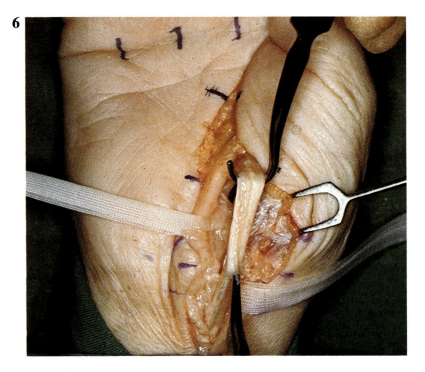

6 A second tape has been passed round the cleaned flexor pollicis longus and the synovium cleaned systematically off each tendon in turn, starting with the index sublimis. A blunt hook can be used to lift and control the tendon, and held by the assistant as the synovium is removed.

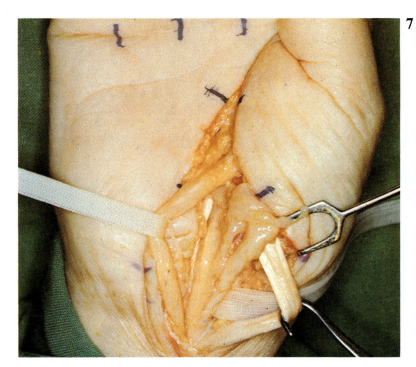

7 The tendon can be pulled proximally and distally by the hook to facilitate clearance along its length. By gently lifting the median nerve it is easy to dissect beneath it along the tendon to the extent of the palmar bursa.

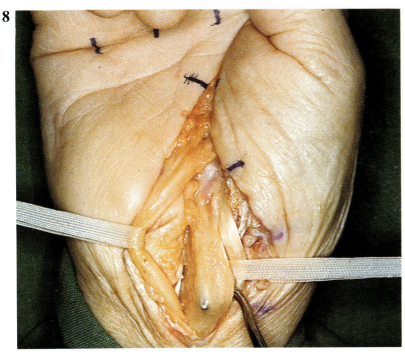

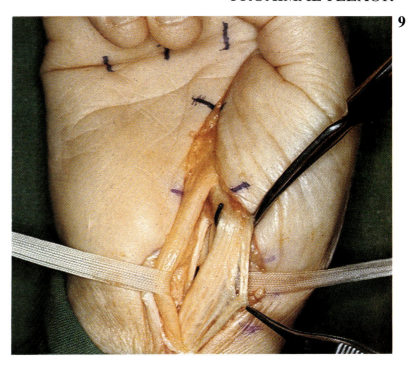

8 As each superficial tendon is cleaned it is taken into the tape and retracted. The sublimis tendons are usually well isolated but the underlying profundus tendons tend to form a bunch as can be seen. Having cleared and collected the sublimis tendons, attention is turned to profundus. In rheumatoid disease these are usually much more affected than the sublimis. They are here lifted to show the matted collection from which by gradual synovial clearance tendons will emerge.

9 The tendons are gradually isolated from the synovial mass. They are often fragmented and show little relationship with the organized system shown in standard anatomical pictures.

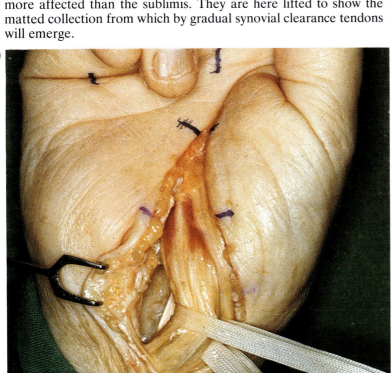

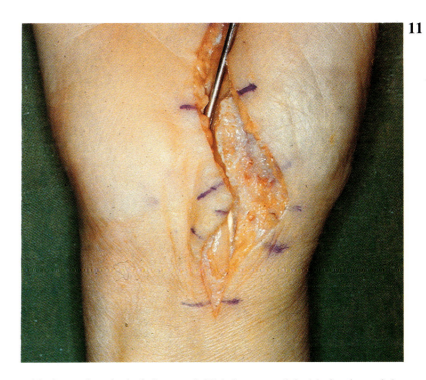

10 Having cleared all the tendons and collected them on the tape, both they and the median nerve should be lifted out of the tunnel and all the remaining synovium removed. Often this is firmly adherent to the surrounding wall of the carpal tunnel and needs to be scraped off. Here it has been removed relatively easily.

11 A suction drain is inserted. This is most advisable in view of the highly vascular nature of the synovium in the field.

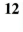

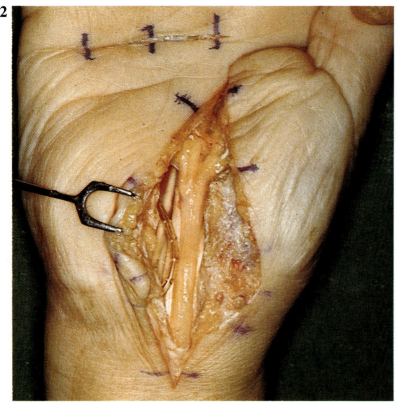

12 The holes in the drain should be well placed in the region of the synovectomy and the wound closed.

N.B. A local distal synovectomy was also carried out on this case, hence the distal incision. Note from this how incisions made in crease lines tend to fall naturally into apposition for easy closure.

Distal palmar synovectomy

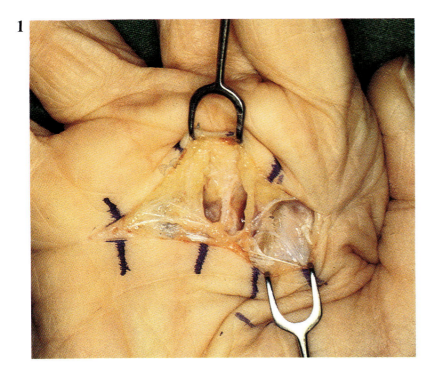

1 The incision is made along the distal palmar crease extending over whichever tendons need clearance – in this case those of the index, middle and ring fingers. The index-finger tendons' mass has been exposed.

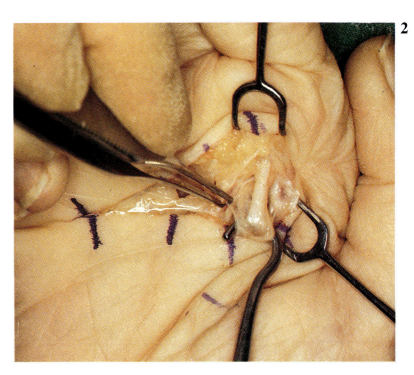

2 A longitudinal incision along the thick synovium allows it to be turned back and a virtually undamaged superficialis (sublimis) tendon lifted by a blunt hook for cleaning, followed likewise by the profundus tendon.

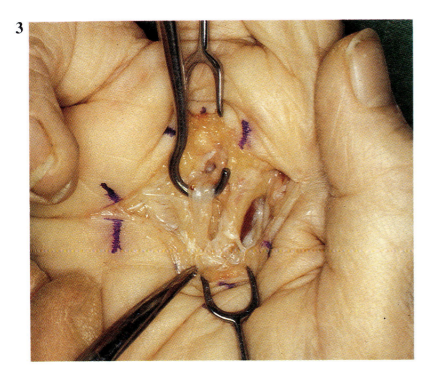

3 The superficialis (sublimis) tendon for the middle finger shows an early tendon granuloma, so far only a surface lesion and easily removable.

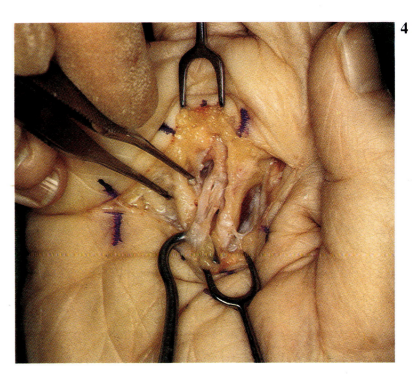

4 When the tendon is pulled proximally from the entrance of the fibrous flexor sheath, after cleaning, a degree of tendon damage may become apparent but limited to this area.

5

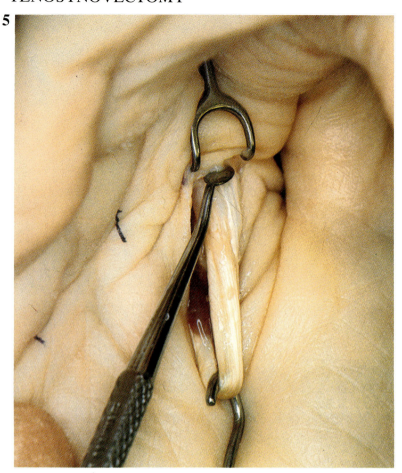

6

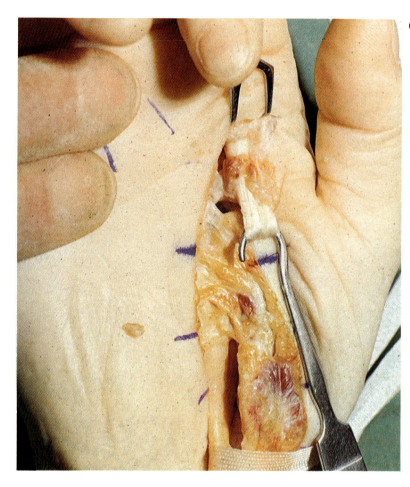

7

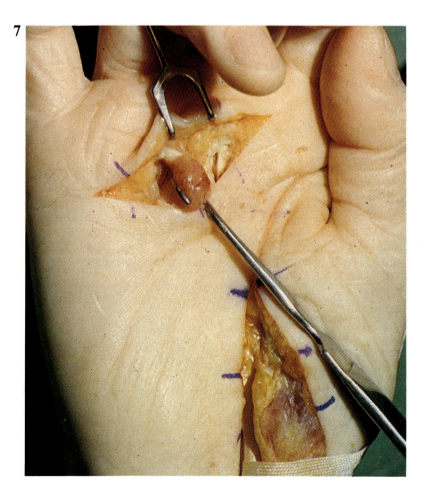

5 Sometimes, as in this case, there is active synovitis at the entrance of the fibrous flexor sheath which can be seen once the tendon has been cleaned. To avoid opening the sheath an adequate clearance can often be achieved by using a Mitchell's trimmer or similar instrument.

6 If the distal tendon clearance is carried out together with a proximal flexor synovectomy the transverse incision may be limited to the ulnar three digits, whilst the index finger can be dealt with from an extension of the thenar crease incision into the proximal transverse palmar crease. The two incisions are thus limited to crease lines, producing minimal scarring in repair, and keeping a stabilizing bridge of skin between them. In the index finger the entrance to the fibrous flexor sheath lies just distal to the incision, which gives excellent exposure. Here the tendon has been cleaned to the fibrous sheath (note the roughened surface). The tendons have now been pulled proximally, so flexing the finger, showing granulomatous material at the entrance to the fibrous sheath and clear tendon beyond; the finger therefore need not be opened.

7 The other fingers are now dealt with through the shorter transverse incision. Again a thick synovial mass is found which, when the tendons are pulled proximally thus flexing the finger, shows its limitation to the proximal region of the fibrous sheath with relatively normal synovium more distally in the finger.

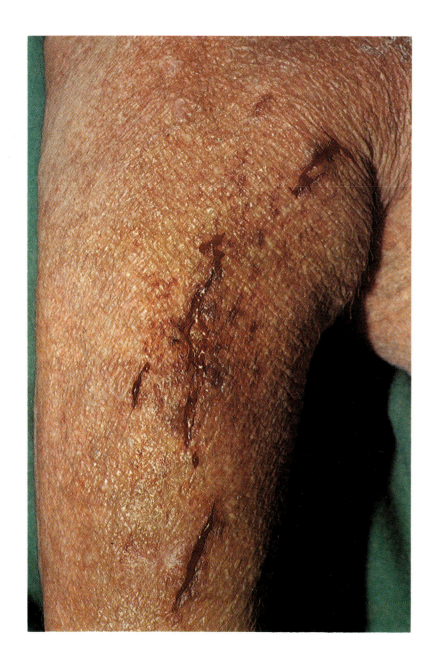

Nearly all the surgical procedures to be described may well be on patients who are or have been, taking steroids. The skin in such patients can be extremely thin and easily torn. Adhesive tape holding the anaesthetist's indwelling intravenous needle can tear off skin flaps unless it is removed carefully.

An Esmark bandage, even when used carefully to exanguinate a limb, can tear the skin as shown here. It is often advisable to restrict exanguination to that achieved by gravity when applying a tourniquet before surgery to a patient who has taken steroids who has severe skin problems and bruising.

SYNOVECTOMY OF JOINTS

6: Synovectomy of the joints

For several years there has been much enthusiasm for early joint synovectomy, before bone erosions have occurred. As stated earlier, the dramatic improvements often prophesized have not been forthcoming. Therefore, the concept of early synovectomy should be broadened to include synovectomy in the later stages of the disease, even after erosions have formed, with the dual purpose of limiting the disease process in that joint before important damage has occurred (the object of early treatment) and to attempt to limit the destructive process at a time when soft-tissue reparative procedures are still possible.

There is no doubt that early synovectomy in a state of a really active and particularly seropositive disease is of little value; the local synovitis usually recurs too quickly and the progress of the disease in the treated joints is likely to continue much as before. However, if the treatment is reserved for those earlier cases in which synovial bulk persists with medical treatment, or when natural remission brings down the disease activity, or both, then the prognosis is far better. Synovectomy is probably more valuable in treating synovial bulk than the disease itself – though it can, if done at the right time, materially influence the progress of the disease in the region.

The problem is deciding when to perform synovectomy and when it is not worth while. In many cases remission will occur either spontaneously or with medical treatment. From Kay's observations the chances of such recovery in the inter-phalangeal joints are far higher than in the metacarpo-phalangeal.

If synovial bulk persists in the joints, the problem of activity against inactivity arises. Whereas digital activity is likely to limit soft-tissue failure (though the bone may suffer more from erosions), inactivity predisposes to soft-tissue collapse with the production of such problems as volar subluxation and ulnar drift at the metacarpophalangeal joints and boutonniere and swan's-neck deformity in the proximal interphalangeal joints. The terminal interphalangeal joints are not usually affected in rheumatoid disease but are commonly affected in psoriatic arthropathy.

Persistent bulk in any of the joints calls for synovectomy, particularly when it remains despite overall disease control. It is often said that synovectomy is a waste of time once erosions have formed. This is true only if the measurements are based on radiographic evidence. Erosions may persist or even grow; they are more likely to do so than to heal. However, the reduced bulk usually leads to better mechanical control and increased power and activity. If the erosions increase this is a relatively small price to pay for the functional improvement but erosions may heal or remain more-or-less static if they are thoroughly cleaned at the time of synovectomy. With increased activity there is also likely to be increased bone density.

The essential feature of synovectomy is that it must be thorough; synovium must be scraped from the inside of the capsule and not just delicately removed. Perhaps the scraping increases the healing fibrosis in the capsule, reduces blood supply for regenerating synovium and thus the risks of rheumatoid reactivation. Whatever the reason, our results have improved since its adoption after a more disappointing phase of performing synovectomy with maximum delicacy. The use of small dental-type instruments such as a Mitchell's trimmer together with a very small spoon help in cleaning out erosions and mosquito-type forceps with the jaws ground out to form micro-nibblers (the ratchets should also be removed) are also very useful.

Metacarpophalangeal synovectomy

The incision is not important as long as there is adequate exposure and care is taken not to disturb the venous and lymphatic channels which run in the groove between the metacarpal heads. A full transverse incision, which is often used, puts these at risk and particular care therefore needs to be taken when using this approach; occasionally there is a tendency for some contraction across the hollow between the heads, giving an ugly cosmetic result. One of the authors (KMB) uses a lazy S, the other (SHH) a straight midline incision to each joint; both give satisfactory exposure and an excellent scar, which in most cases becomes almost invisible. A longitudinal incision is recommended in the extensor expansion. The value of making this incision to the radial side of the extensor tendon – rather than along it – is that it allows easy plication with overlap of the expansion at the region where it is most likely to be stretched, and for this reason it is most commonly practised. The joint is said not to have a capsule dorsally but there is usually a certain amount of fibrous material representing a thin capsule between the extensor expansion and the synovium. This fibrous material may be thickened in rheumatoid disease. This material should be divided longitudinally and preserved, as it is often useful as additional support to the expansion in the repair. If the operator does not know of its presence it will be removed with the synovium.

The thick synovium will now be found; it may be fleshy and bulky or thinner and filled with thick synovial fluid material including solids; sometimes, particularly after treatment with gold, the synovium is fibrous. The activity of the disease can often be gauged by the synovial vascularity. The synovium will commonly be found extending a considerable distance proximal to the joint. If this is grasped first and pulled distally the synovium can then be separated from the dorsum of the metacarpal head. The collateral ligaments should then be identified. In a severely swollen joint the synovium may well overlap them dorsally or be adherent so that they are often not easy to find, especially if they have become thinned and stretched. Some operators divide one or other of the collateral ligaments so as to dislocate the finger laterally, thus giving better access to the volar aspect of the joint. However, this is not our practice. We proceed to separate the synovium from beneath the collateral ligaments and then divide its attachment to the base of the proximal phalanx. The attachment to the phalanx is often quite thick and fibrous, especially in a patient taking gold. If the joint is now taken into full flexion and distracted, fine mosquito nibblers can be slipped into the volar aspect of the joint and the synovium at the proximal end of the volar plate removed. Care should be taken to clear all the synovium beneath the collateral ligament and it is here that erosions are likely to be found. The granulation tissue and synovium should be removed from these as efficiently as possible and it is here that dental instruments are particularly useful. If erosions are thoroughly cleaned out they will often heal; if not they will inevitably progress.

The extensor expansion can now be repaired. It will be noted that the expansion is asymmetrical in that the more dominant ulnar side interosseous muscle has a much thicker attachment to the extensor tendon than the radial. Thus the thinnest part of the expansion over the metacarpophalangeal joint is a triangle to the radial side of the extensor tendon (Backhouse 1968). Hence this is the part of the expansion most likely to be stretched and thinned by the disease with the eventual disloca-tion of the extensor tendon into the gutter between its own and the adjoining metacarpal head. In repairing the extensor expansion it is useful to overlap the expansion by plication to allow take up of the stretched portion and to return the extensor tendon to its original position if at all displaced. However, the major displacement cannot be repaired simply by plication. Some form of soft-tissue realignment will be needed; either a relatively simple procedure done with a synovectomy as in pages 187 to 191 or a more extensive one as in pages 182 to 186.

The suture material for the expansion should be chosen with care. A material such as silk will become embedded in fibrous tissue which shows as unsightly nodules through the skin; even the black may be seen if that colour of silk is used in a patient taking steroids. Dexon and Prolene are useful materials, the Dexon being absorbed.

A similar approach can be made to the thumb metacarpo-phalangeal joint. In the case of the thumb there is much to be said for extension splinting for a period postoperatively, as stretching of the expansion of this joint commonly leads to fixed flexion deformity; splinting in extension in the early healing phase may allow some take up of the stretched extensor aponeurosis and so reduce the tendency to flexion.

Metacarpophalangeal joint synovectomy

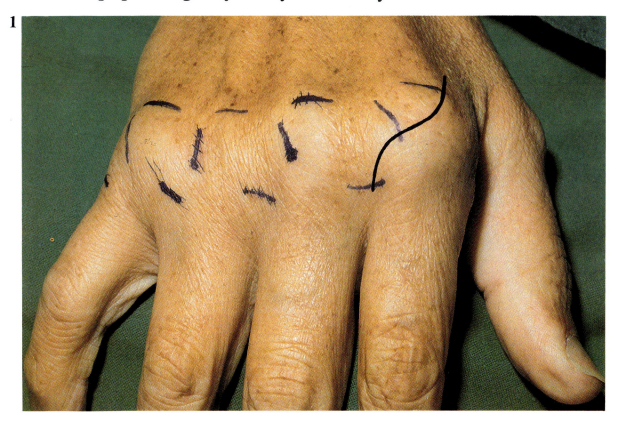

1 Relocation marks are made on the skin to assist in accurate re-suture of the lazy S incision. The incision line has been super-imposed on the index joint. If a straight midline incision is used, marks are unnecessary.

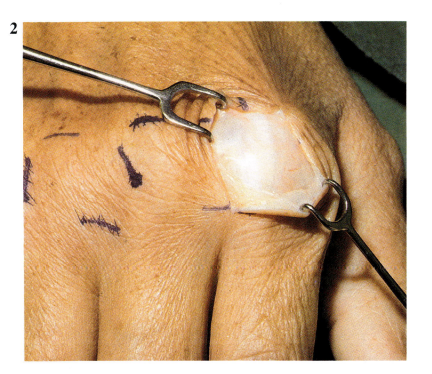

2 The extensor expansion is exposed. In this finger there is only small ulnar displacement of the tendons.

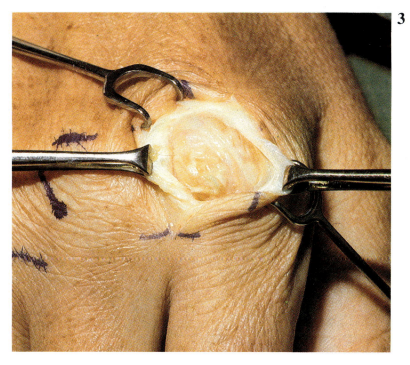

3 The expansion is divided longitudinally to expose the thick, fleshy synovium. If the expansion is held by such small-toothed clips as the Allis variety skin retraction can be discarded and good access controlled to the synovium.

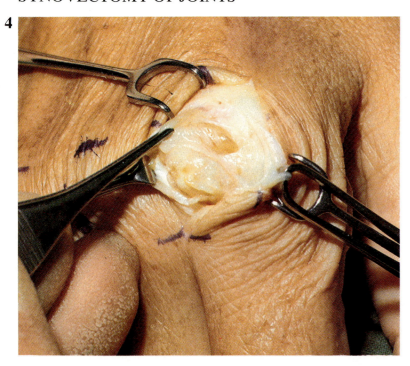

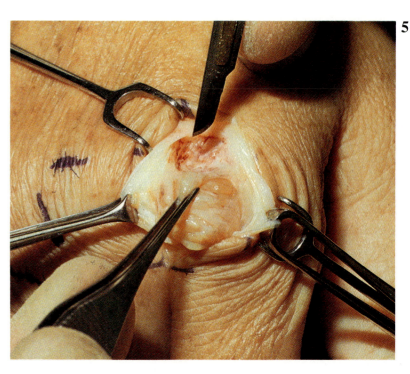

4 The synovium can now be grasped firmly and pulled distally to free its proximal extension. The material often tracks a considerable distance proximally under the expansion; far more than would be expected from normal anatomical descriptions.

5 The proximal mass of synovium can now be separated from the bone; usually sharp dissection is needed. The damaged hyperaemic metacarpal shaft to which the synovium had become adhered is now exposed and the normal attachment line of the synovium to bone at the cartilage edge is found.

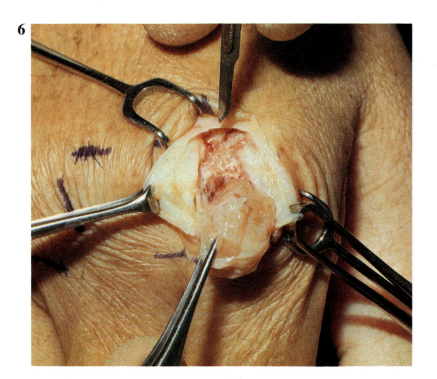

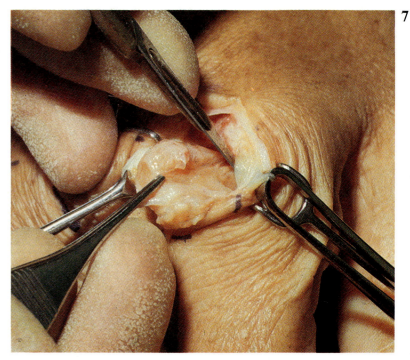

6 The synovial mass is now divided from the metacarpal attachment dorsally.

7 The collateral ligaments should now be identified. This may not be easy, especially if the ligaments are stretched and thinned or the synovium shows some fibrosis. The ligament is often firmly adhered to the synovium and needs to be separated by sharp dissection. Here identification is easy and the synovium is being cleaned from the deep surface of the ligament, and then the bone deep to the ligament.

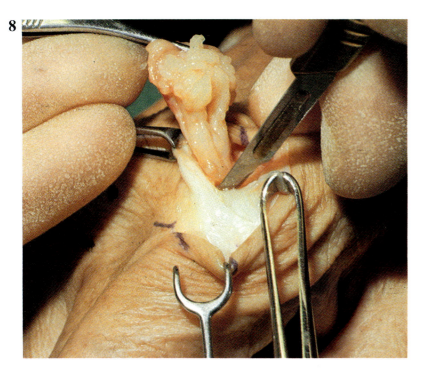

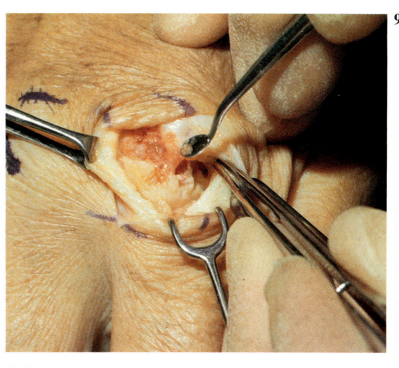

8 When the collateral ligaments have been cleared the synovium is cut from the bone of the proximal phalanx. There may be fibrous attachments of the extensor expansion here which should be left if they remain intact despite the synovial damage.

9 Erosions, particularly beneath the collateral ligaments, need to be cleared of granulation tissue. An erosion pocket can be seen here beneath the ligament, having been cleared with a Mitchell's trimmer (or similar dental instrument).

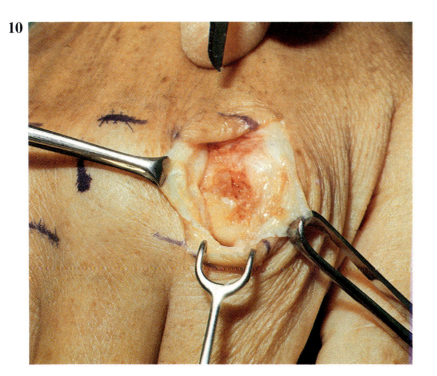

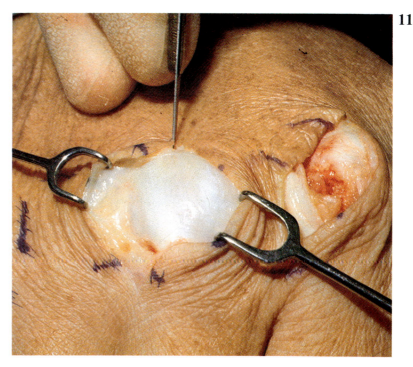

10 The joint has now been cleaned dorsally and fine mosquito forceps have been pushed through to the volar aspect to drag out material alongside the volar plate, leaving a clean, though eroded joint.

11 The next joint can now be approached. In this case the extensor tendon shows considerably more dislocation and stretching of the expansion to its radial side than in the case of the index finger.

12

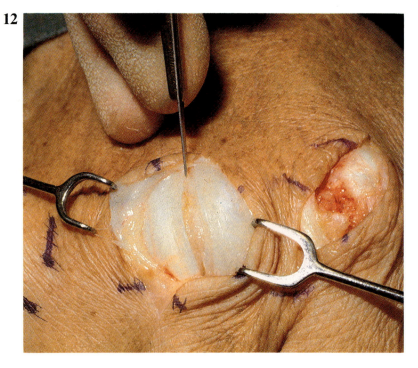

13

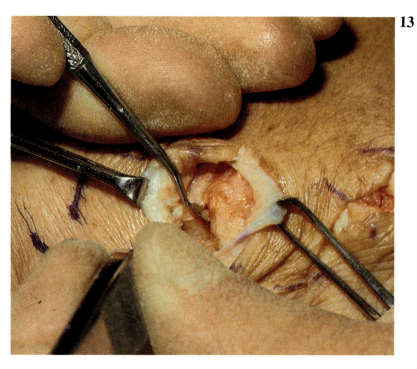

12 The operation proceeds for each finger in turn as shown for the index.

13 In each joint careful toilet of bone erosions is most important.

14

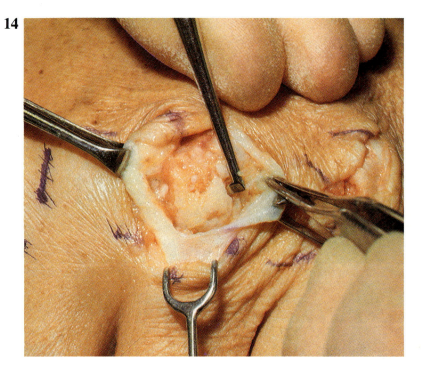

15

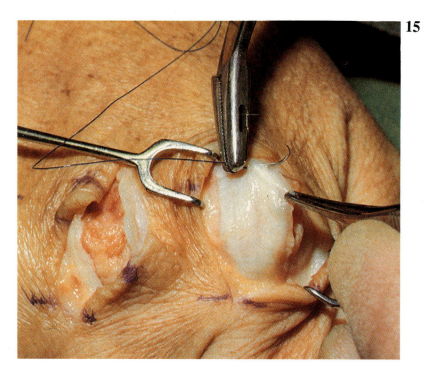

14 Sometimes erosions are quite deep despite appearing to be quite small superficially. Here the sharp end of a Mitchell's trimmer is almost filling the pocket, some 4–5 mm deep.

15 Repair of the expansion can be done immediately but there is an advantage in waiting until the adjoining joint has been cleared, especially if there is likelihood of carrying out muscle realignments. In this case it was decided that a satisfactory simple repair could be achieved. A stitch is therefore put through the extensor tendon.

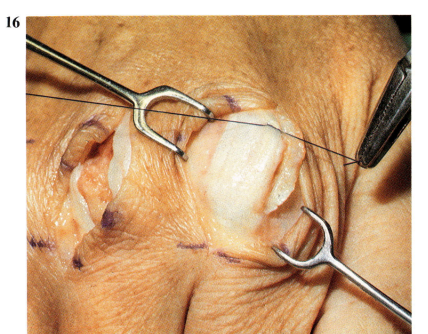

16 From the surface of the tendon the needle is now passed through the radial side of the extensor expansion and the radial collateral ligament and tied. This is repeated more distally so that the extensor tendons are correctly sited and anchored to the radial side.

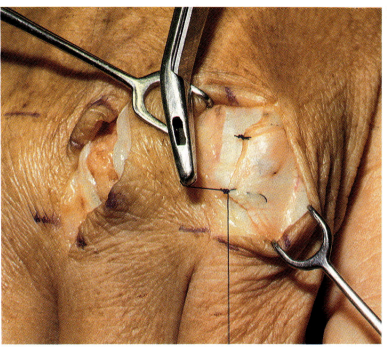

17 The spare stretched radial expansion is now stitched across to overlap the extensor tendons. In this case Dexon has been used as the suture material.

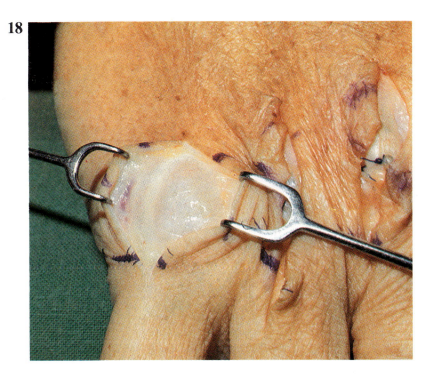

18 The little finger shows considerable ulnar displacement of the extensor tendon, together with ulnar drift of the digit.

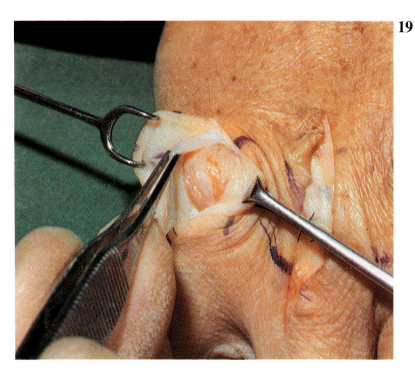

19 The clearance proceeds in the same way as the other fingers.

20

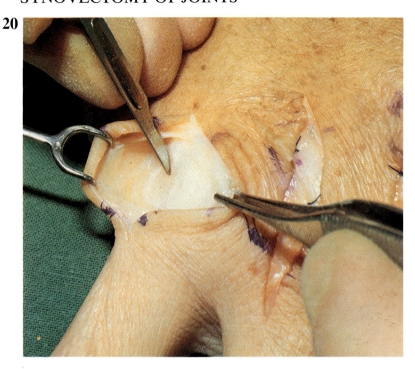

21

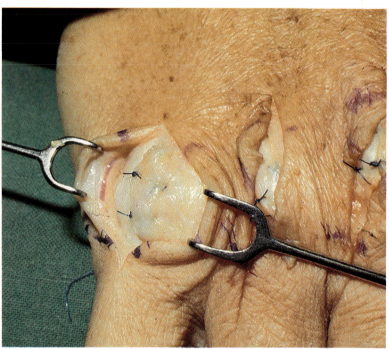

20 The extensor expansion is now divided longitudinally to the ulnar side of the extensor tendon to allow it to be pulled radially. This is satisfactory only if the abductor digiti minimi is still not showing the shortening which will occur in longer standing cases of drift and the fingers can easily be moved radially.

21 The expansion is now repaired as the other fingers, giving good position to both tendons and finger.

22

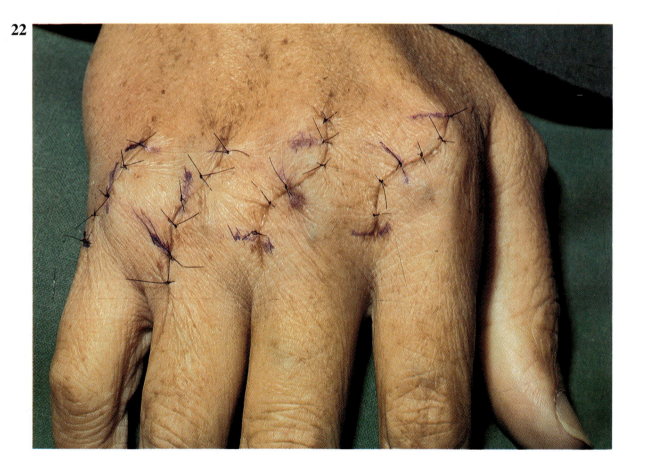

22 The wounds can now be sutured. Using such an incision there is excellent exposure and a beautiful scar can be expected.

Metacarpophalangeal synovectomy of the thumb

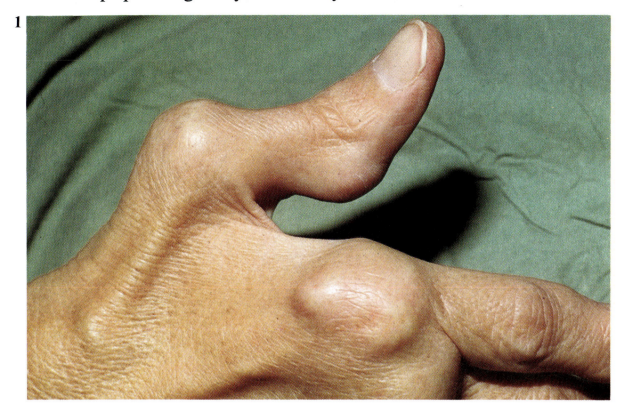

1 Synovial thickening in the thumb commonly produces stretching of the extensor expansion. The extensor brevis tendon insertion may be stretched or pushed aside: as is the case for extensor pollicis longus, and the insertion of the thenar muscles into the expansion disorganized as shown here. The joint falls into fixed flexion with a compensatory hyperextension of the interphalangeal joint, which then also becomes fixed.

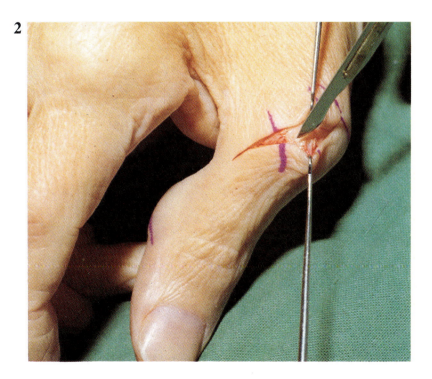

2 Synovectomy is likely to be of value only while the joints are still mobile. A lazy S incision is used here to expose the stretched expansion.

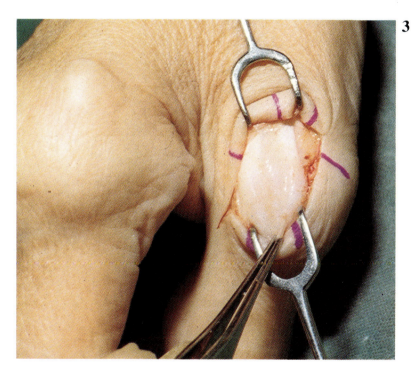

3 The expansion shows the extensor tendons one to each side of the joint. The thinned expansion between is divided longitudinally.

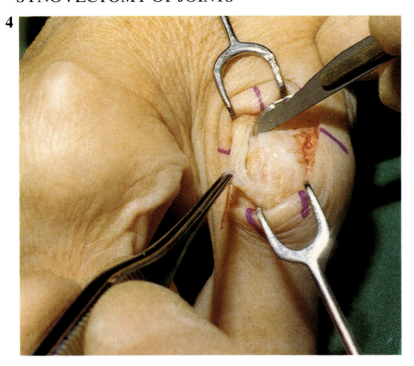

4 The adhered expansion is dissected from the underlying synovium and taken laterally.

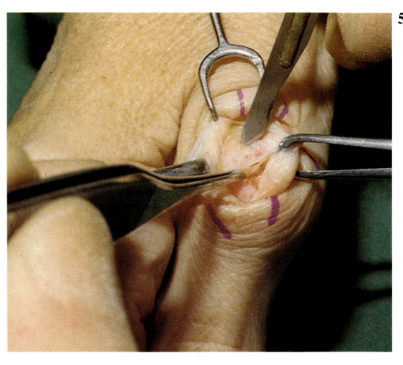

5 The synovium is lifted proximally and dissected off the metacarpal head, carried distally and cleared from the remaining joint structures.

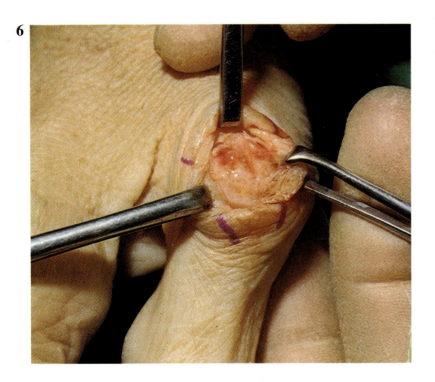

6 The bone shows erosions which need to be cleaned thoroughly of granulation tissue.

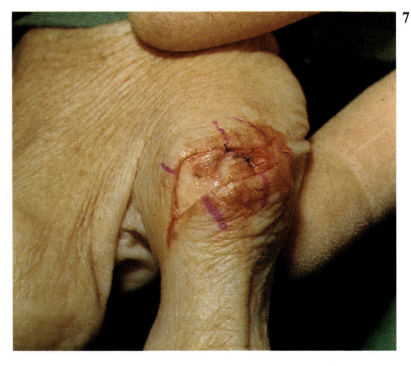

7 The expansion is resutured with overlap to produce an effective anatomical positioning of the tendons; the extensor pollicis brevis tendon may be shortened if necessary.

8

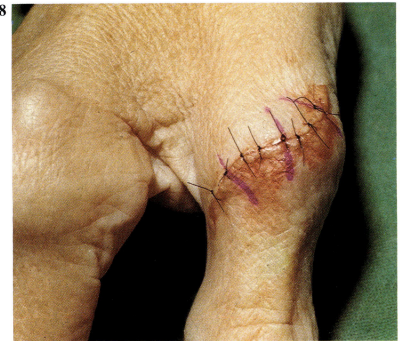

8 The wound is sutured and the joint set up in extension with a little interphalangeal flexion, if this is reasonably possible, for the wound-healing phase.

Synovectomy of the proximal interphalangeal joints

This differs from that of the metacarpophalangeal joints, mainly because of the difference in the extensor expansion.

A similar incision can be used over the dorsum to that for the metacarpophalangeal joints but it is often advisable to approach the volar aspect of the joint as well as the synovial vincular extensions to the tendons. A triple-curved incision is always used by one of us (SHH) which allows the dorsal approach to the joint and also a lateral approach to the volar aspect from the same incision.

The extensor expansion can be divided by two incisions between its three component bands, or it can be detached from one side and turned backwards across the finger to get to the synovium. Its removal can proceed most effectively from proximal to distal as in the metacarpophalangeal joints. The only difference is that in the double dorsal incisions through the expansion the synovium must be taken in halves from the two sides. The volar aspect can then be approached to a small extent through the joint but more effectively by dividing the glenoid ligament between the collateral ligament and the volar

plate and so reach the volar synovium. This last material is sometimes relatively large in amount and effect in this joint and can play an important part in establishing such problems as swan's-neck deformity and joint fixation.

Occasionally in rheumatoid disease but more often in psoriatic arthropathy the distal interphalangeal joint may be helped by synovectomy. This can be approached dorsally, taking care to limit the incision to avoid the nail bed. The extensor tendon can be retracted to allow approach to the synovium and then repaired with some advancement, as the tendon is often stretched over the joint.

In synovectomy of the interphalangeal joints it is advisable to set the finger in extension postoperatively at these joints to allow some extensor tendon support and take up and to reduce the occasional risk of flexion deformity. The extensor aponeurosis is usually quite severely stretched over the joints before synovectomy is carried out in the interphalangeal joints. Hence, when the bulk is removed the finger falls forward into flexion which can, if not corrected early, become permanent.

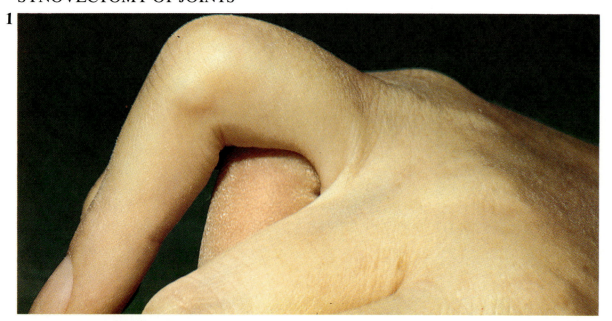

1 The swelling of the joint can be seen, and the proliferating synovial tissue has extended out of the joint beneath the intrinsic tendon on the radial side.

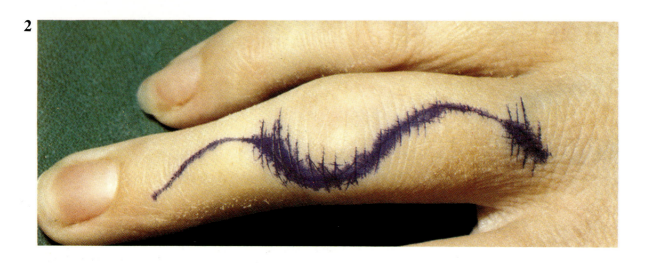

2 A triple-curved or three-flap incision was designed so that the dorsum and anterior compartment of the joint could be exposed through one incision.

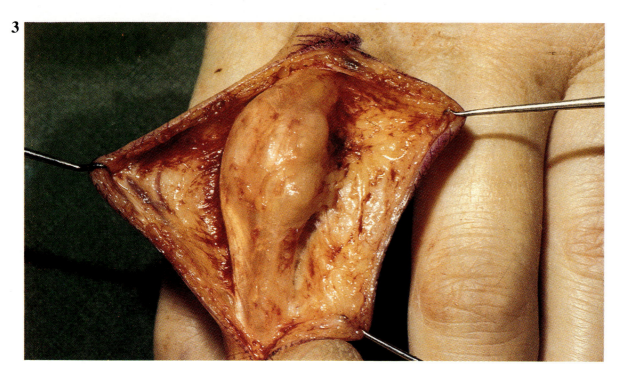

3 The extensor tendons are exposed and the mass of proliferating tissue can be seen bulging out of the joint beneath the radial intrinsic tendon.

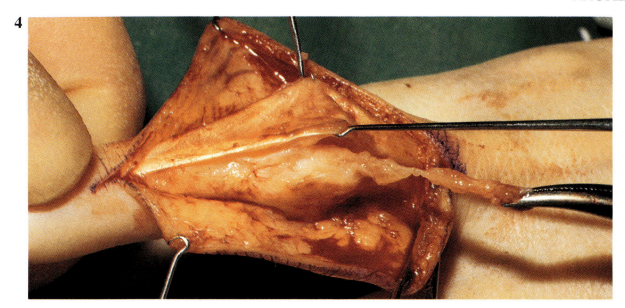

4 An incision is made on both sides of the joint along the anterior margins of the intrinsic tendons. The synovial tissue is passed beneath the extensor tendon from the medial to the lateral side and removed.

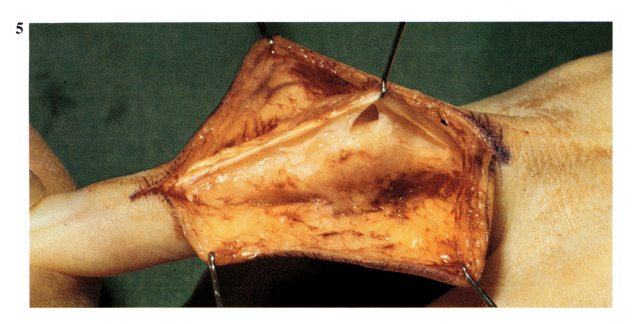

5 The extensor on the radial side has been raised with a skin hook, and the interior of the joint inspected.

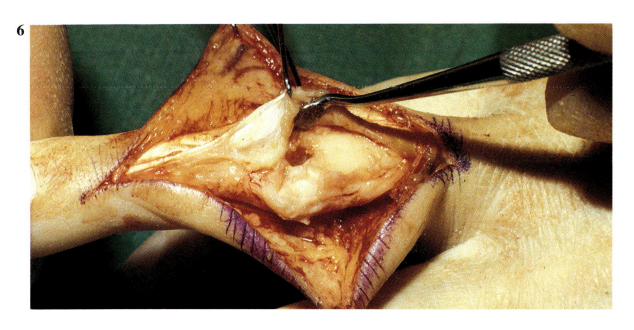

6 An erosion in the bone has been exposed on the radial side of the head of the proximal phalanx, affecting the attachment of the collateral ligament. This is curetted with a Mitchell's scaler. In some cases this procedure can affect some healing, as later radiographs often show sclerosis of the margins of the erosion.

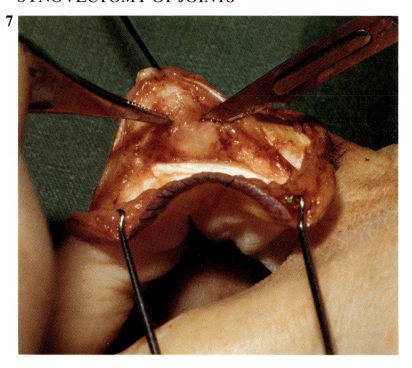

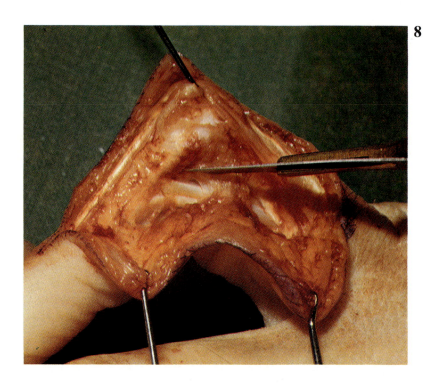

7 The anterior compartment of the joint is exposed, and the upper margin of the volar plate defined.

8 The anterior compartment of the joint is opened by an incision along the upper margin of the volar plate.

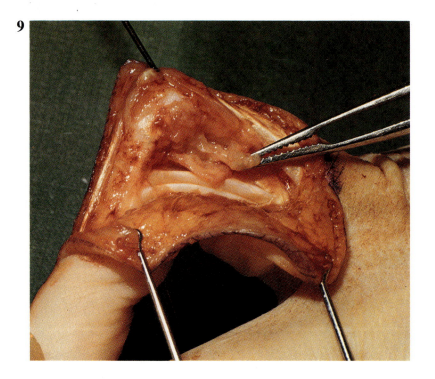

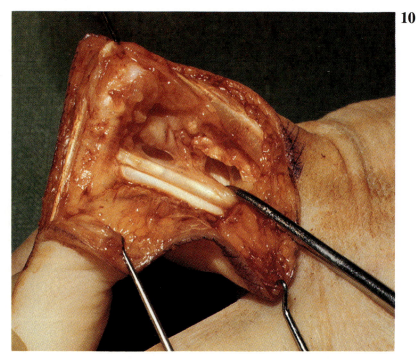

9 A mass of proliferating synovial tissue is removed from the joint.

10 The flexor tendons are retracted, exposing the check ligament which can be seen to have been affected by the proliferation of synovial tissue. The flexor tendons should be inspected to ensure that there are no nodules present, which might interfere with movement, and any proliferating tissue adhering to the tendons removed.

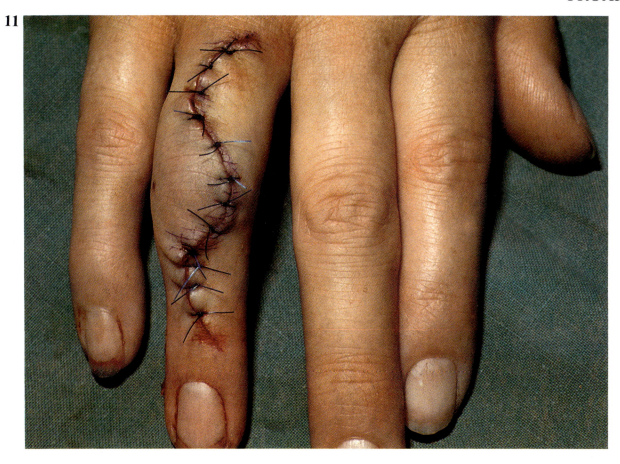

11 The tourniquet is released and the wound closed. A dressing is applied, and the hand elevated. The next day the bandage and dressings are removed and a single piece of sterile gauze is wrapped around the finger. Movements are started and the patient advised to adopt a regimen of intensive exercises for 10–15 minutes in every hour. Full movement should be regained in 10 days, when the sutures are removed.

Synovectomy of a digital proximal interphalangeal joint (2)

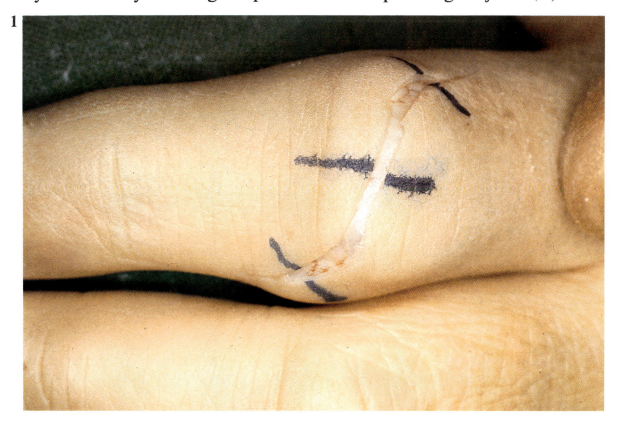

1 Skin relocation marks are made with a sterile pen and a lazy S incision made. This should extend to the sides of the fingers to give at least lateral approach to the joint and the volar plate. The advantage of this incision is that it makes maximal use of the crease lines but is a less good approach to the palmar aspect of the joint than the triple-curved incision shown on page 86.

2

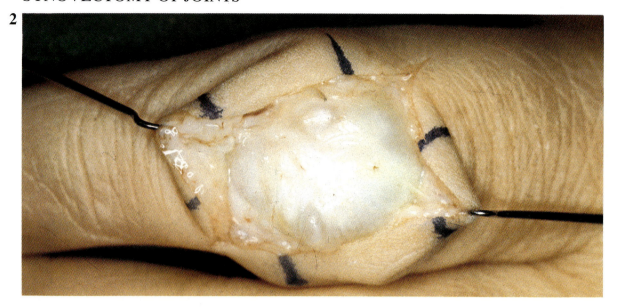

2 The skin flaps are separated and retracted to expose the extensor expansion. Here small herniations can be seen between the central and lateral slips of the expansion. This tendon disruption is one important criterion for carrying out a synovectomy of this joint.

3

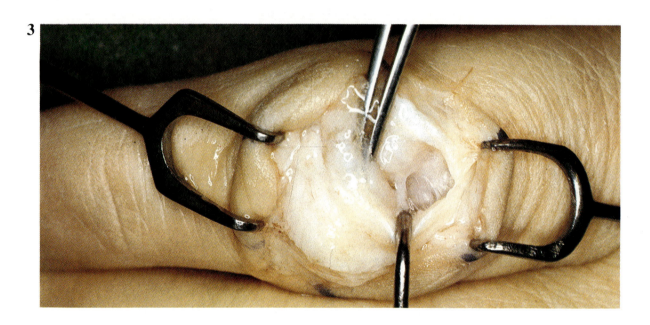

3 Incisions are made between the medial and lateral slips (i.e. in the region of the herniations). The synovial material is removed on each side through those incisions. The synovium is pulled distally from the proximal end and separated from its bone attachment, then between bone and collateral ligaments and finally separated distally.

4

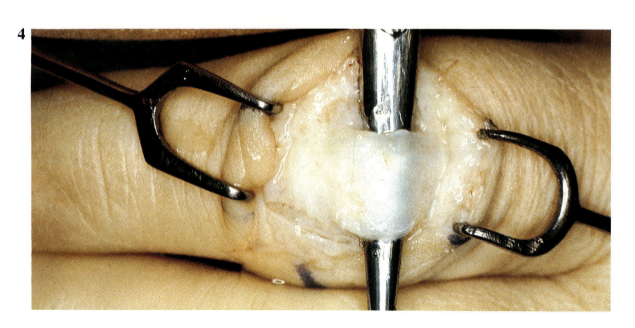

4 Most of the material is now clear, leaving usually a somewhat lax stretched central slip of tendon.

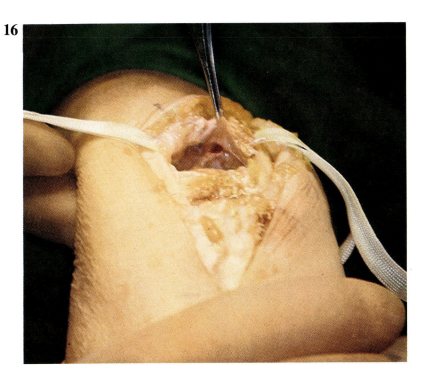

16 The distal end of the radius is, in this case, a mere shell with a cavity extending 2 cm up the bone. After cleaning out it healed well and the patient was left with a virtually painless, stable wrist with adequate mobility.

Excision of the head of the ulna (ulnar styloidectomy)

There is often considerable damage and distortion to the distal end of the ulna, with relatively little extensor tenosynovitis. This may occur in rheumatoid disease or other inflammatory arthropathies as a relatively isolated synovitic lesion, as a sequel to one of these diseases with superimposed osteoarthrosis, or from osteoarthrosis alone.

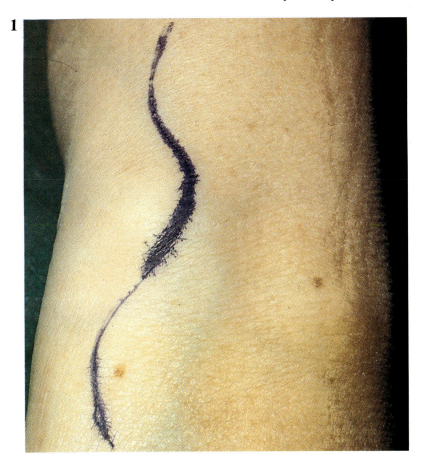

1 A triple-curved (flap) incision (SHH) is made over the dorsum of the ulnar head. (A short transverse incision along the wrist crease as wide as the ulnar head and then turned proximally along the ulnar border is also used by some surgeons (KMB).

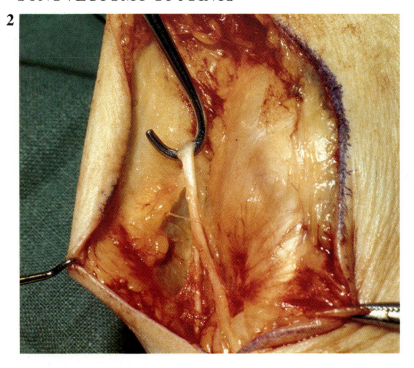

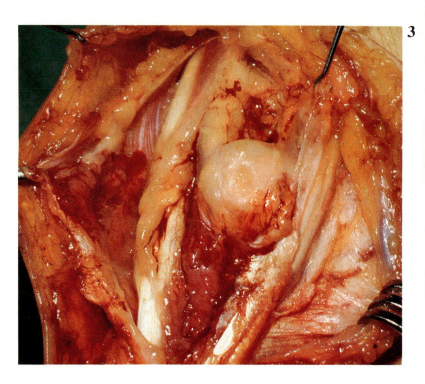

2 The dorsal cutaneous branch of the ulnar nerve comes off the main trunk, 5 cm above the wrist joint, and then curves around the ulnar head. This branch should be dissected clear from the field.

3 The capsule of the joint is opened dorsally. The eroded head of the ulna can be seen lying between the extensor carpi ulnaris and the extensors of the ring and little fingers.

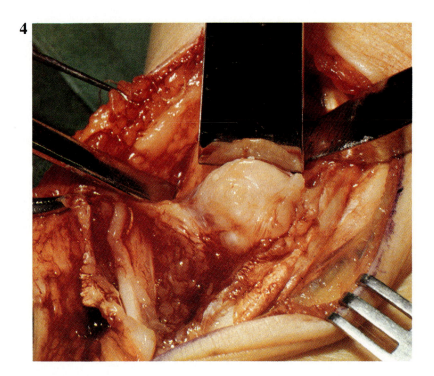

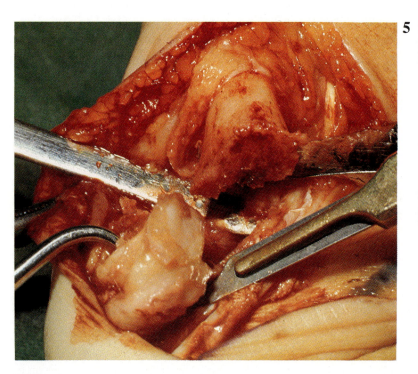

4 The head of the ulna has been cleared of soft tissue. A rugine has been passed beneath the bone to protect the soft tissue anteriorly from the osteotome, which is used here for sectioning the bone.

5 The head is held with a sharp hook and is removed by sharp dissection.

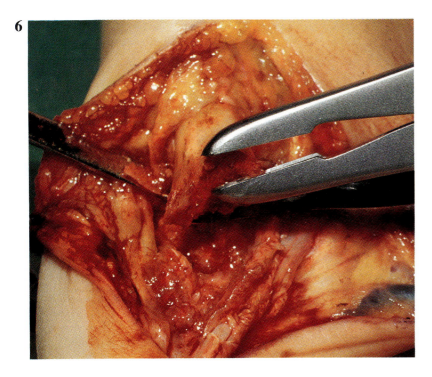

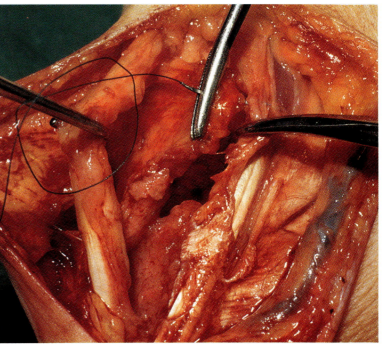

6 It is important to round off the proximal end to eliminate any sharp edges, which might damage adjacent tendons. It is also important not to remove any more of the head than is necessary, otherwise there will be pain on pronation and supination, owing to whip of the uncontrolled bone end, and the extensor tendons may be at risk from the whip of the bone.

7 The distal end of the ulna should be covered with soft tissue of the capsule, leaving the digital extensors free from their sheath on the radial side. The tourniquet is released and the wound closed. Postoperatively, a Zimmer splint may be incorporated in the bandage until the sutures are removed. Further splintage may be required if there is pain on pronation and supination, in which case the splint should be worn at decreasing intervals until the wrist is free from pain.

Synovectomy of the proximal radio-ulnar joint

As for the distal radio-ulnar joint, this is difficult to carry out effectively without removal of the head of the bone – in this case the radius. Occasionally, simple synovectomy is worth considering, especially if there is some elbow instability and it is combined with synovectomy of the elbow joint and there is no important damage to the radial head. But this type of synovectomy is difficult to perform effectively and should be considered only when there is fleshy synovium causing mainly capsular stretching in an otherwise medically controlled case. If, however, the elbow is in a reasonably good state and there are important bone changes to the radius, then it is unwise not to remove the head. A reasonably stable elbow will result and an adequate synovectomy of the joint is possible. Only the head of the radius need be removed to clear the annular ligament and the joint surface with the ulna.

The posterior interosseous nerve passes onto the neck of the radius after transversing supinator muscle in about 60 per cent of cases. In rheumatoid disease in particular but even in osteoarthritic change of the joint the supinator may be small in bulk because of disuse atrophy; the large synovial mass may well have extended distally to a considerable extent and the posterior interosseous nerve may be stretched over the synovium to be removed and can very easily be damaged.

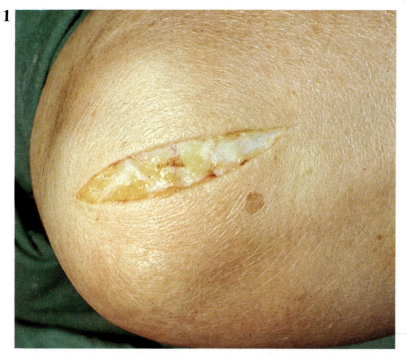

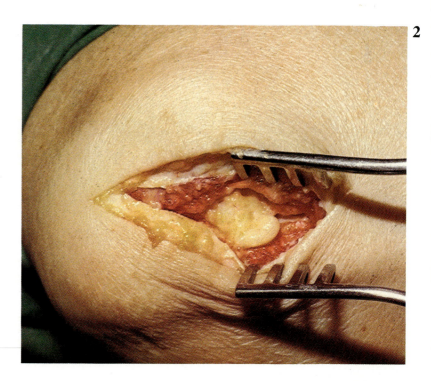

Synovectomy of proximal radio-ulnar joint with excision of the radial head

1 A longitudinal incision is made over the radial head dorsally. This should run distalwards from the level of the tip of the olecranon to the level of the neck of the radius.

2 The muscle is separated from the side of the olecranon to expose the dorsal aspect of the joint. Commonly there is fat between muscle and joint.

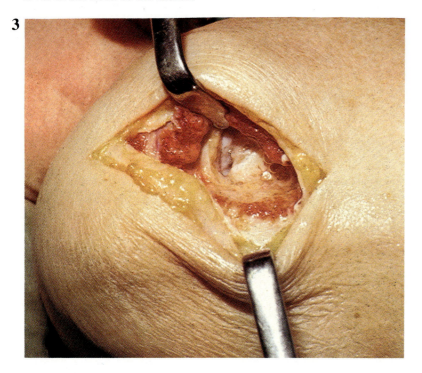

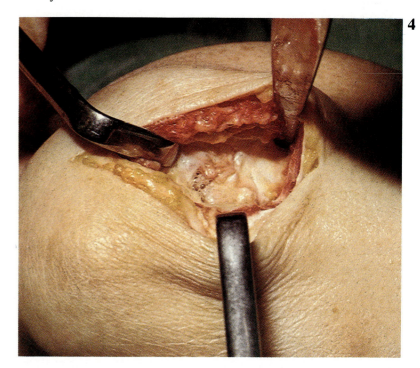

3 The dorsal capsule of the joint is divided longitudinally. The annular ligament can be seen around the radial head.

4 The dorsal synovium can be removed at this stage to expose the bone. A bone spike can be used to control the radius.

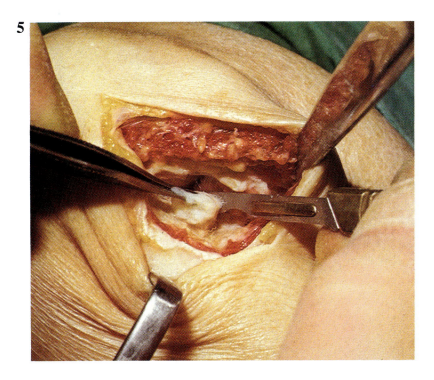

5 The annular ligament is also divided dorsally to free the radial head.

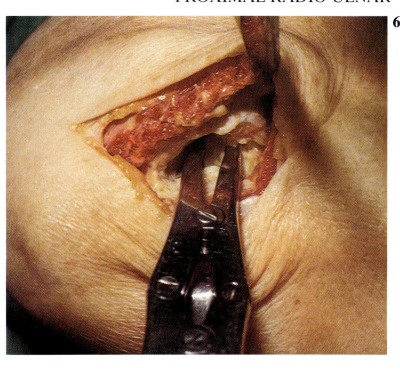

6 The method of excision must depend upon the surgeon's own preference. In rheumatoid disease, however, the bone is relatively soft and often grossly mis-shapen. There is therefore much to recommend the use of bone nibblers. Small pieces of head are removed initially.

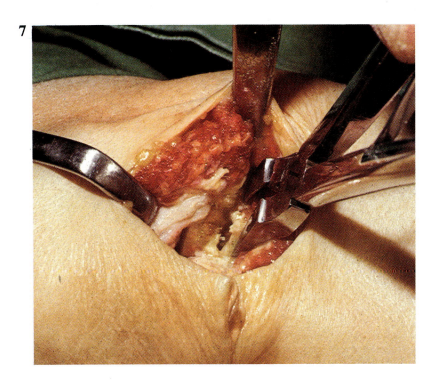

7 The neck of the bone can be identified and cut through once the rough overhanging bone has been removed.

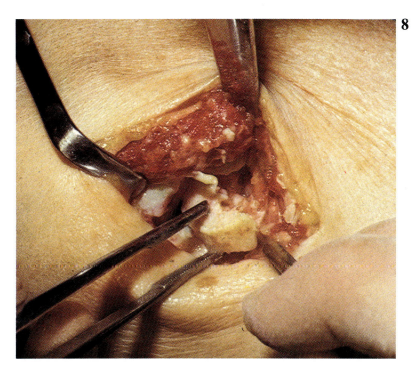

8 The head is now separated from the shaft and ligamentous attachments divided.

9

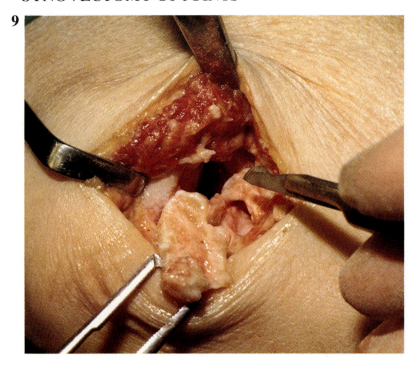

9 As the distorted head is removed the thick synovium can be seen in the depths of the joint.

10

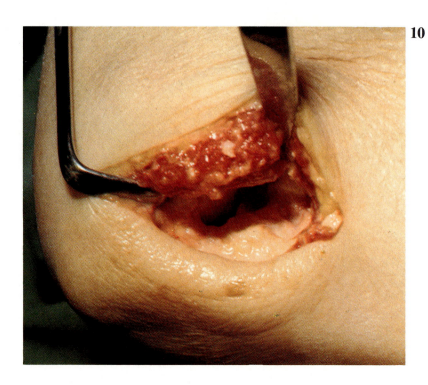

10 The synovium can now be removed leaving a clean joint capsule. Care must be taken in this process to watch for the posterior interosseous nerve. It may lie on the neck of the radius and, particularly if it has become stretched by the thick synovium of the joint, it can far too easily be pulled up into the vicinity of the operation field.

11

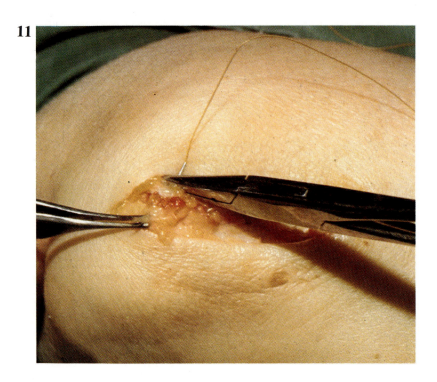

11 The dorsal capsule is now repaired.

12

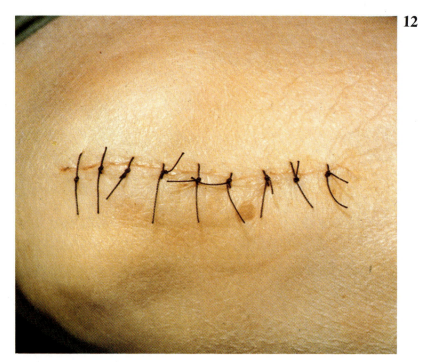

12 Followed by the skin.

Synovectomy of the elbow joint

This is also not easily carried out effectively, since the proximal radio-ulnar joint is bound to be affected. As stated above, removal of the radial head may be advisable but there may be reasons for its retention. It is often said that the olecranon must be removed for an effective synovectomy. This is probably true, but it must be replaced postoperatively either by lag screw or wiring; this seems a drastic procedure to give a slightly more

complete clearance of a joint than may be otherwise achieved. The recurrence rate may be higher without removing the olecranon, but the difference is not so great that the problems of the bone repair in a diseased joint can be neglected. We find that an adequate synovectomy and good results can often be achieved with the simpler procedure.

If there is gross increasing instability of the elbow joint but without proximal radio-ulnar joint damage it is reasonable to limit the synovectomy to the elbow joint itself. An adequate exposure can be achieved by a bilateral approach, though it must be appreciated that

the radio-ulnar joint cannot have a satisfactory clearance. Removal of the olecranon with later replacement gives a better approach but is far more drastic and not necessary.

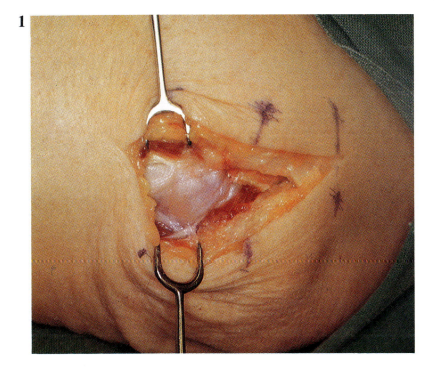

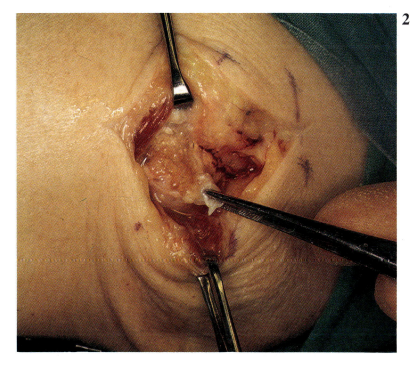

1 The first incision is made to the radial side of the olecranon. This gives a good approach to the elbow joint above supinator and the posterior interosseous nerve.

2 The joint capsule is opened behind the radial collateral ligament and the thick synovium removed from the dorsal aspect of the joint.

3

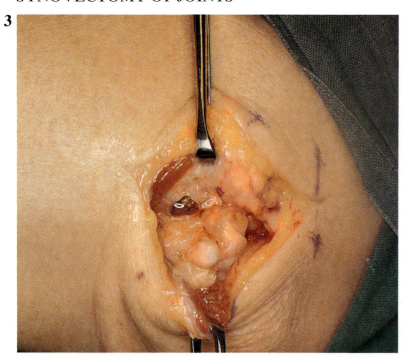

4

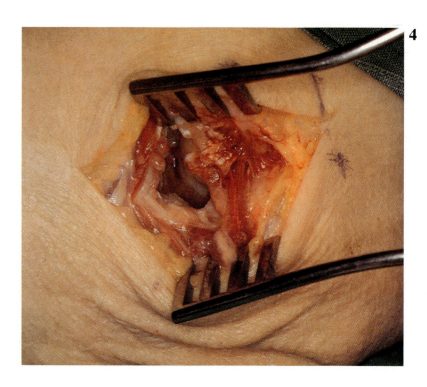

3 The bone can now be cleaned. Not infrequently free bodies – sometimes 'melon-seed' like material – are to be found in the joint, as shown in this picture.

4 Because of the laxity of the ligaments the bones can often be distracted enough for an approach to the volar aspect of the joint and the proximal radio-ulnar joint. However, as here the radial collateral ligament can be divided a few millimetres away from the lateral epicondyle. Only the posterior fibres normally need to be cut. The joint can now be opened more easily.

5

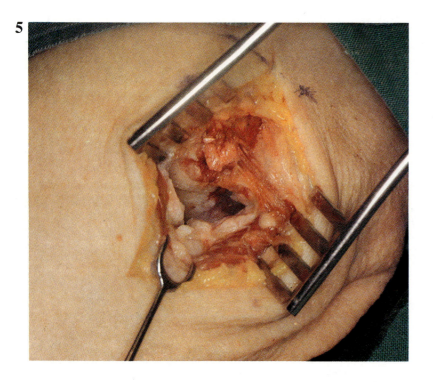

6

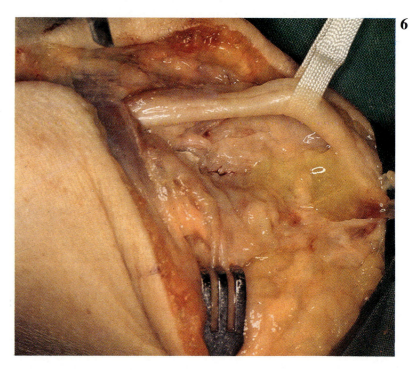

5 The periarticular erosions can be cleaned out. The collateral ligament can now be repaired and attention switched to the ulnar side.

6 A much longer incision is required on the ulnar side than the radial as the ulnar nerve has to be mobilized. Care must be taken to look for the branches of the ulnar nerve; to the elbow joint (which is usually lost) and particularly to flexor carpi ulnaris. Here the first branch runs into the muscle near to the joint and therefore mobilization of the nerve had to be limited. Usually it can be freed to the full length of the skin incision.

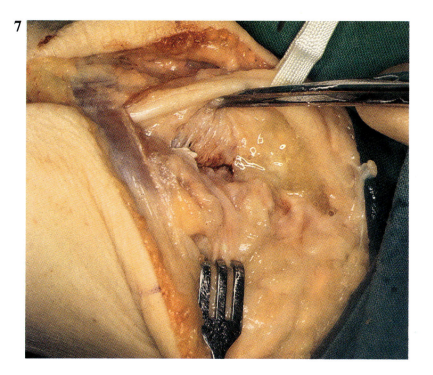

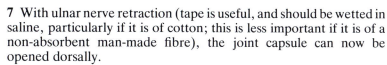

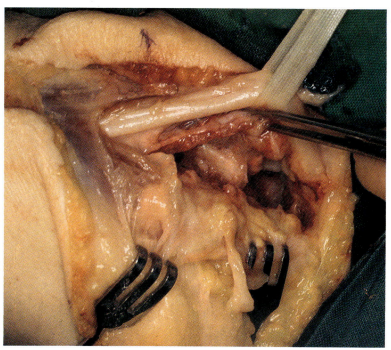

7 With ulnar nerve retraction (tape is useful, and should be wetted in saline, particularly if it is of cotton; this is less important if it is of a non-absorbent man-made fibre), the joint capsule can now be opened dorsally.

8 Synovial clearance is now possible. Again distraction may be all that is necessary if the ulnar collateral ligament is lax but division, particularly of the posterior band of the ligament, can be helpful. The ligamentous structures are repaired and the skin sutured. Care must be taken to limit any lateral stress during the healing phase (3 weeks or so). This will often allow ligamentous take up, particularly if supported by suturing. In this particular case a very swollen painful joint with severe lateral instability was essentially painless, stable and useful 2 years later.

TENDON REPAIR

7: Tendon repair

Reparative and reconstructive procedures are the methods of repair used for the rheumatoid hand in which tendons or ligaments have ruptured and joints displace or subluxate from erosive change. The object is to produce functional rehabilitation of the affected part.

There is likely to be a chain reaction, in which one deformity leads to another: for example, flexion deformity of the thumb metacarpophalangeal joint will lead to hyperextension of the terminal joint; or ruptured extensor tendons if neglected may allow subluxation to occur at the metacarpophalangeal joints, and subsequently a repair of the tendon will have to be associated with a reconstruction of the joints.

It is necessary to recognize these potential liabilities early and to intervene surgically at a stage where the progress to deformity can be effectively interrupted.

Reconstruction is mainly concerned with the early correction of joint alignment before the deformity has become established, at which stage only salvage by arthroplasty or arthrodesis can effectively restore the basic elements of function.

Tendons may rupture from various causes. Rupture is usually said to be because of attrition over bone spicules or a hypermobile ulnar head, but far more commonly in rheumatoid disease the site is away from such possibilities. From our studies it would appear far more likely, in most of cases, to be caused essentially by hydrostatic pressure changes where bulky synovium is pulled into the confining spaces of retinacular tunnels. Whatever the cause, before the tendon ruptures there will be bundle fragmentation and necrosis over a considerable length of tendon. There will also be change in the physical structure of the collagen. Hence there will always be a length of tendon lost and what tendon remains will inevitably have disrupted and necrotic ends which will need to be excised before repair is possible. End-to-end suture will therefore rarely be possible and it is necessary to use either grafts to bridge the gap, other tendons with their muscles switched to take over, or the ruptured tendon joined to another comparably functioning tendon to give a mass action.

In rheumatoid disease further ruptures may take place later and prodigality in the use of materials is undesirable. The results can never be expected to be as good as in a clean incised wound, for instance; nevertheless, as with so much of surgery in the arthritic conditions, it is important to think of giving functional improvement and control of the disruptive processes rather than a 100 per cent cure. Also, the tendon rupture has probably not occurred in isolation and it will be one of several problems in a disorganized hand. Thus in choosing the method of repair it is important to think of the overall hand function before and after surgery, the possible future developments of the disease and even the changes in mechanics brought about by the repair.

The extensor tendons are the most likely to rupture, particularly those to the thumb and little finger, and then possibly in sequence to the other fingers but this is less likely. In the palm, although tendon damage is very common, tendon rupture is less common than might be expected. However, if it does occur it is a serious disability and often occurs in the so-called 'no-man's-land' of tendon surgery, at the distal end of the palmar bursa or in the finger. One other problem of tendon repair is that whereas traumatic cases are likely to arrive at a casualty department and be available for early treatment, the rheumatic patient tends to be treated at a slow pace via the next appointment with the rheumatologist and a further wait for a surgical appointment as a 'cold' case. Muscles will by this time have become contracted and atrophic.

There is a wide range of possibilities for repair, remembering the gap between normal tendon which usually prevents end-to-end anastomosis. The obvious method is tendon graft using palmaris longus, a short toe extensor, or possibly plantaris. This is the method of choice in no-man's-land in the palm but in the rheumatoid state other methods can reasonably be used. It is often possible to split the proximal part of the ruptured tendon and use this as a bridge graft, either as a simple graft or as a reflected bridge graft (SHH) as shown in **Figure 7.1**. A method which is extremely useful but for some reason rarely practised is to slide the proximal part of the tendon from within its muscle fibres and to re-attach it to the muscle far enough distally to allow end-to-end suture of the tendon. The disadvantage of the technique is its technical difficulty of maintaining control of the muscle fibres after

7.1 As an alternative to splitting a tendon and excising a piece completely for use as a bridge graft, the end of the tendon can be secured from splitting by fine sutures and the split portion turned back on itself and sutured to the other tendon end. Hence a small blood supply may be retained at one end of the bridge, thus increasing the chances of survival.

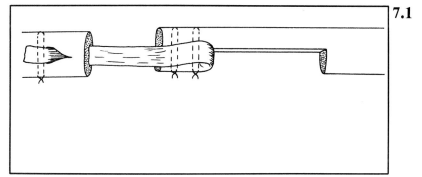

7.1

separation from the tendon ready to re-attach, but this can be achieved easily enough if the sutures are applied to the muscle before separating it from the tendon. One of us (KMB) uses this technique occasionally, and finds it very satisfactory.

Another common method is to switch an adjoining tendon which is regarded as of relatively subsidiary importance to take over as the motor. Often if mass action gives an adequate result – and this may be far more acceptable in the rheumatoid state than in the more normal hand – the ruptured distal end may be joined to an adjoining tendon, so sharing its muscle; the ruptured proximal end may also be attached to give pull from both muscles through one tendon.

Whatever is done for the tendon repair it is essential to carry out an effective tenosynovectomy first. If other tendons are

also badly damaged it may be advisable, especially if it is some time after tendon rupture, to anchor the ruptured ends and carry out the repair some weeks after synovectomy, by which time much repair of the damaged tendons will have taken place and it will be easier to assess the best way of repairing the rupture.

Sometimes a tendon may have become denatured and stretched, or even after rupture a bridge of tissue composed of paratenon and synovium which has become fibrosed may bridge the tendon ends. In both these states in extensor tendons the stretched material can simply be plicated. If the hand is held in extension initially on a splint for 3 weeks followed by lively splinting, allowing active flexion, the end results may be comparable with a graft.

Rupture of the extensor pollicis longus

The commonest tendon in the hand to rupture is the extensor pollicis longus, and rupture is often preceded in rheumatoid disease by the appearance of synovial proliferation around the proximal part of the tendon on the dorsum of the hand. This should have been an indication for earlier prophylactic synovectomy.

Not infrequently the patient may be unaware of the rupture; merely of reducing function. Rupture may occur with or without trauma.

The rupture is diagnosed by holding the thumb fully extended proximally and the terminal joint will evidently be in flexion and cannot be extended actively.

In the rheumatoid hand destructive changes are often seen on a radiograph of the first metacarpophalangeal joint. When these changes are present, it is desirable to stabilize the joint at the same time as the tendon is repaired. We use a Harrison-Nicolle intramedullary peg, but arthrodesis by crossed Kirschner wires can be used.

Direct continuity cannot be provided in the repair of the tendon, and tendon transplantation is normally the treatment of choice.

In traumatic or post-traumatic cases, the extensor indicis proprius is often used as the motor tendon, but in the rheumatoid hand it is preferable to use an alternative such as the extensor pollicis brevis. This tendon is excellent because it lies close to the extensor pollicis longus, and therefore requires less dissection, but mainly because it extends the thumb with slight abduction, rather than adduction into the plane of the hand, as occurs when using the extensor indicis proprius transplant (Harrison). This alteration in the plane of extension is important, as one of the primary deformities of the thumb is adduction deformity owing to the carpometacarpal joint being affected, and this should be avoided whenever possible, as will be described later.

Backhouse prefers to make use of the fact that abductor pollicis longus usually has two and sometimes three tendons of insertion, which usually separate back into the muscle. One of the tendons is divided at its insertion for use as the extensor motor of the thumb, leaving the other tendon in its normal insertion. It is also in the same plane as extensor pollicis brevis and hence has the same advantages.

Repair of extensor pollicis longus and arthrodesis of a thumb metacarpophalangeal joint

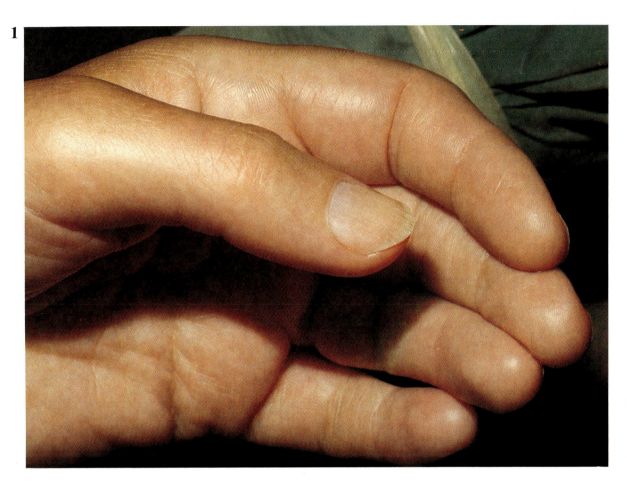

1 The hand is relaxed in the position of rest. The thumb is adducted into the plane of the palm. The thumb is rotated and opposes the fingers. Slight flexion of the terminal joint in this position indicates a long-extensor rupture.

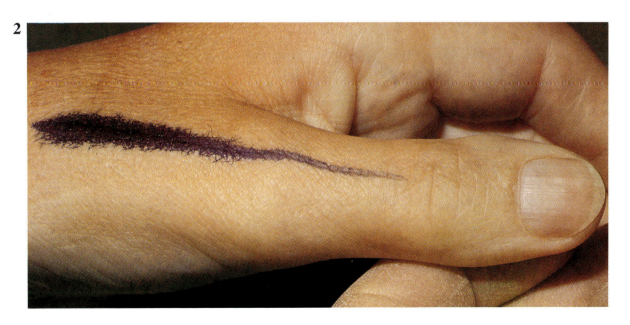

2 A longitudinal incision 5 cm in length is made over the dorsum of the thumb, with the centre of the incision overlying the first metacarpophalangeal joint.

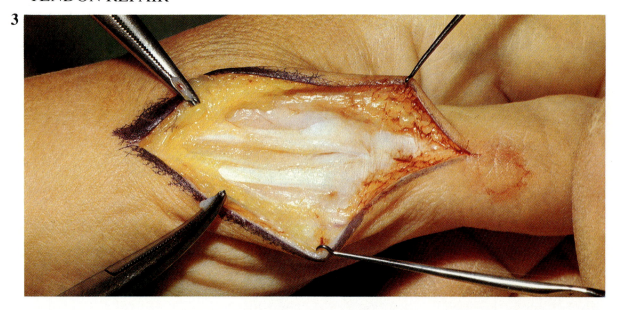

3 This skin is dissected off the underlying tendons and it is essential in this procedure, as it is in all hand surgery, to have a dry field, by the use of a tourniquet, and to use magnifying glasses or binoculars, so that the small branches of the radial nerve can be seen and avoided. The extensor pollicis longus and brevis can be seen lying in the wound. There is a slight corrugation in the extensor pollicis longus, which indicates there is 'slack' in the tendon.

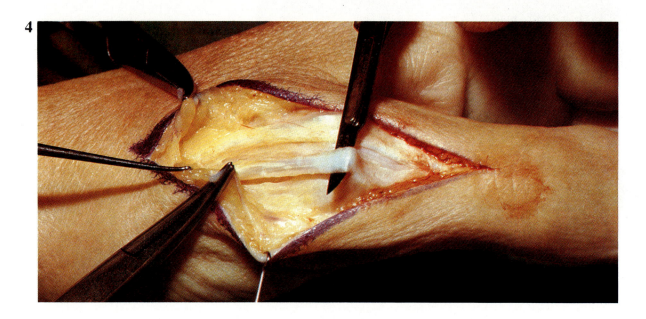

4 The extensor pollicis brevis is divided distally after separating the tendon from the surrounding tissues.

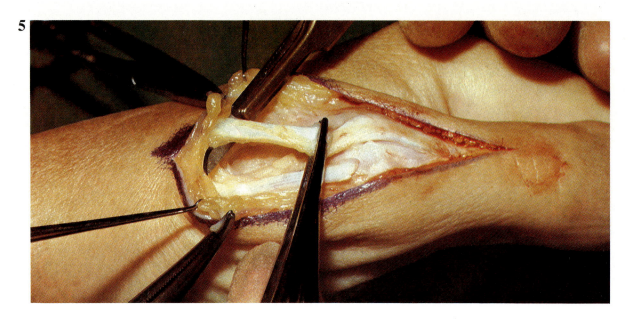

5 The extensor pollicis longus is divided in the proximal part of the wound.

6

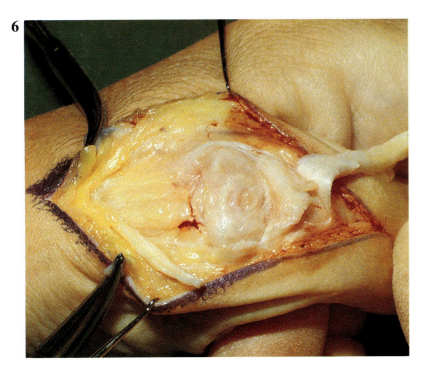

6 The divided tendons are distracted respectively, proximally and distally, revealing a joint capsule distended by proliferating synovial tissue and showing a central necrosis.

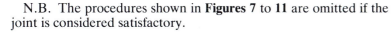

N.B. The procedures shown in **Figures 7** to **11** are omitted if the joint is considered satisfactory.

7 The joint capsule and underlying synovial tissue is excised. A sharp bone-hook is inserted into the articular surface of the base of the proximal phalanx for distraction. The articular surfaces can be seen to have lost some of the cartilage, especially on the superior surface of the metacarpal, partly from erosion and partly from loss of function, as a result of progressive flexion deformity of the joint. This is a characteristic finding in rheumatoid arthritis.

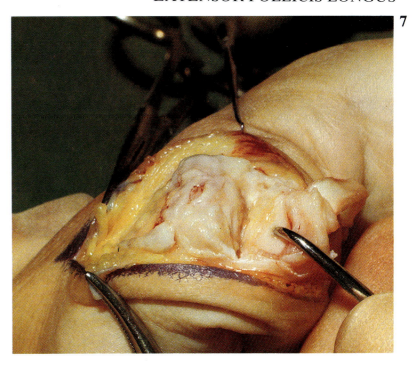

8

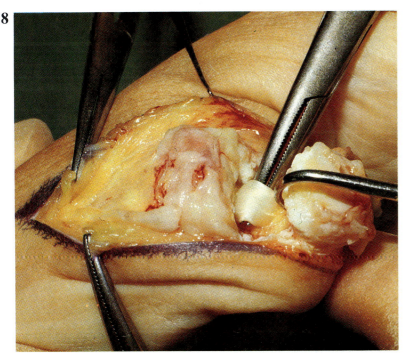

9

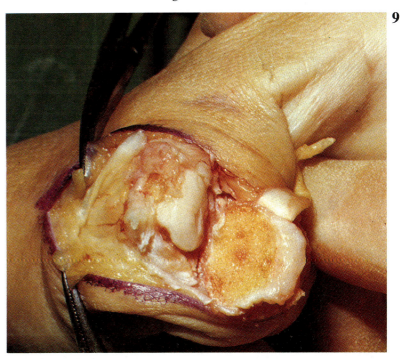

8 The ligaments have been divided and the sharp hook is moved from the articular surface to the anterior lip of the proximal phalanx, making it possible, by distraction, to inspect the flexor tendon which can be seen raised by an artery forceps. This procedure is to confirm that the tendon is in continuity and not invaded by synovial tissue. A large erosion can be seen on the head of the metacarpal.

9 Having freed all the soft-tissue attachments from the base of the proximal phalanx, the articular surface is removed with a chisel, saw, or bone nibblers to obtain a flat surface.

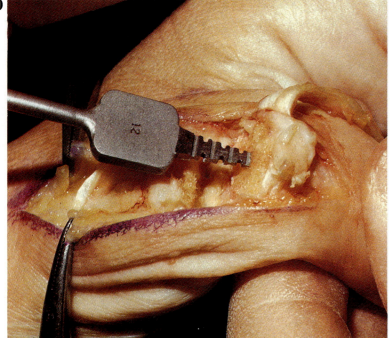

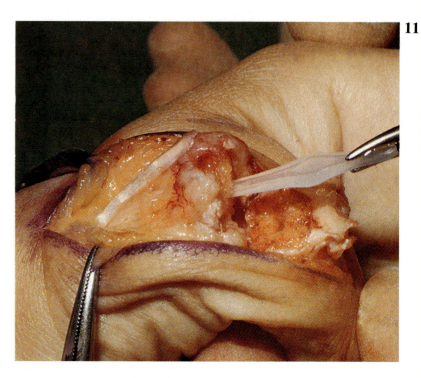

10 A small perforation is first made in the centre of the base of the proximal phalanx, and this is followed by the insertion of the distal end of a Nicolle reamer. The reamers are graded, and have a distal and proximal end similar in size to the stems of the Harrison–Nicolle polypropylene pegs. A number 6 reamer will make a suitable hole to accommodate the straight peg. The procedure is repeated for the head of the metacarpal.

11 The bone surfaces should be shaved flat, so that they are in close contact, and should be so designed that after fixation the thumb will have 15–20° of flexion, pronation and radial angulation at the junction. The straight peg is first inserted into the metacarpal, and then the distal end is inserted by fully distracting the base of the proximal phalanx with a sharp hook in the anterior lip.

The junction is now impacted by compression to eliminate any gap and the dorsal capsule closed.

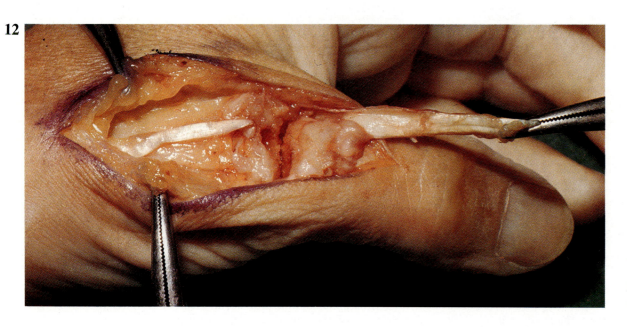

12 The completed bone junction is shown with the peg in situ. The extensor pollicis longus is held distally and the extensor pollicis brevis can be seen in the proximal part of the wound.

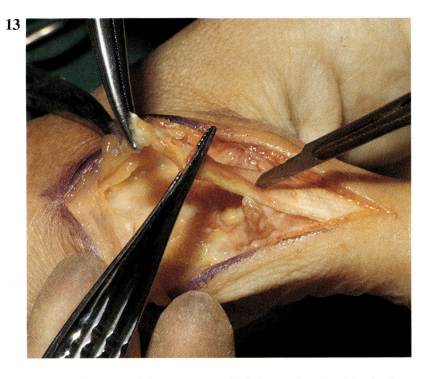

13 The distal end of the extensor pollicis longus is split with a knife. The proximal end of the extensor pollicis brevis is then passed through the split.

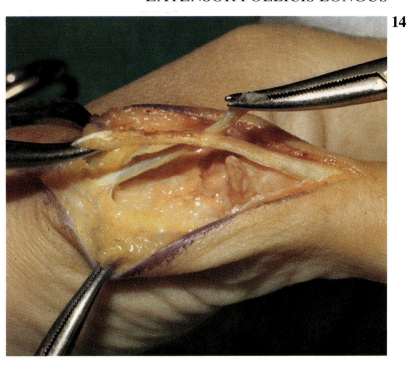

14 Both tendon ends are held taut, and at this stage the thumb is held fully extended with the terminal joint in hyper-extension.

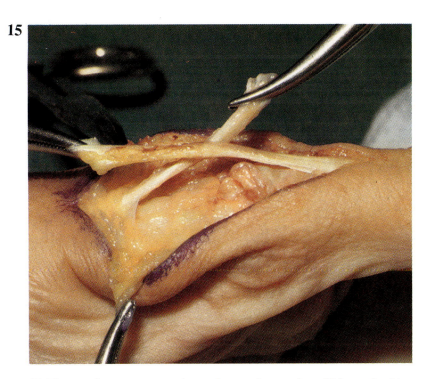

15 The tendons are sutured together under tension. This method is called 'the button-hole technique'.

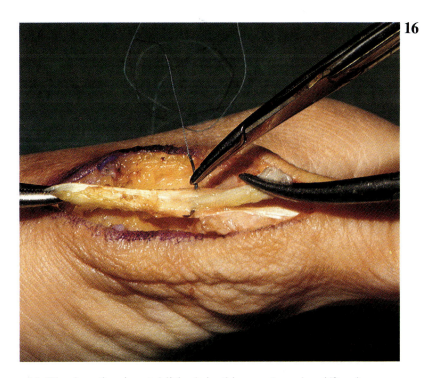

16 The junction is established, in this case by using 4/0 nylon on a small, curved, cutting needle.

17

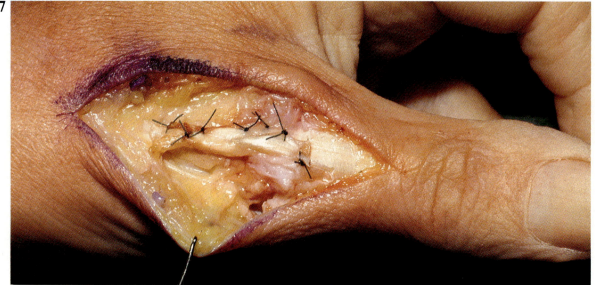

17 The loose tendon ends are removed and the short ends sutured to the underlying tendon. The final junction can be seen.

18

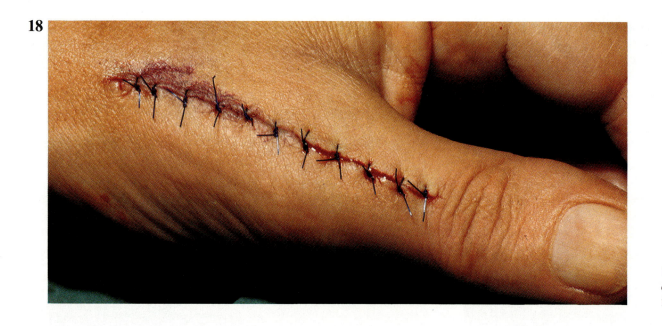

18 The skin is sutured and plaster of Paris is applied with the thumb in extension.

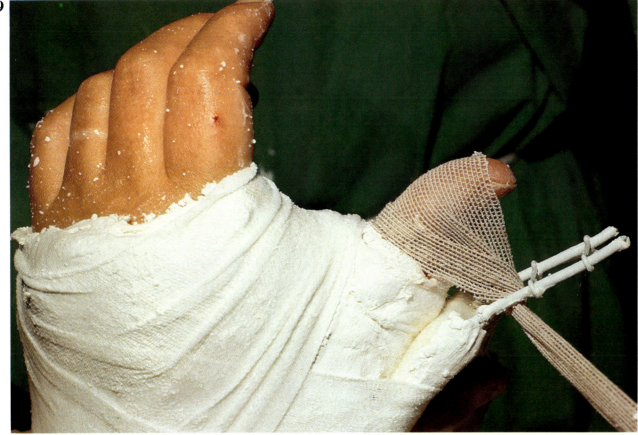

19 It is advisable in rheumatic cases to insert a 2.5 cm wide Cramer wire splint into the plaster of Paris, as an outrigger, and attach the terminal phalanx to this with a leather cuff or sling, via a rubber band. Alternatively, this can be done with an elasticized material such as Lastonet. This allows the patient to exercise the terminal joint without jeopardizing the tendon junction. If this is not done in rheumatic cases there is a risk of stiffness in the terminal joint occurring after 4 weeks' immobilization.

N.B. If abductor pollicis longus is used as the motor the junction will need to be made more proximally over the carpometacarpal joint because of its shorter length.

Rupture of the digital extensor tendons

After the thumb the extensor tendons to the little finger are the most likely to rupture.

Occasionally, the extensor digiti minimi tendon ruptures within its sheath of paretenon, and appears intact until the thickened sheath is opened to expose either an empty sheath or a reconstituted tendon consisting of fibrous tissue.

The next commonest tendon to rupture after the little-finger tendon is the ring-finger tendon, followed by that of the middle finger. The extensor of the index finger seldom ruptures individually, but follows rupture of the above three, with or without an intact extensor pollicis longus.

After rupture of an extensor tendon of a digit in a rheumatic patient, the hand should be splinted in a reasonably extended position as soon as possible after the rupture has occurred, otherwise the other extensor tendons may follow. Furthermore,

if the digit is not splinted or the tendons repaired immediately, and there is concurrent metacarpophalangeal disorganization, the base of the proximal phalanges may subluxate on the head of the metacarpal, and then it will not be possible to repair the extensors, unless the subluxated joint is corrected at the same time. If there has been considerable delay, then arthroplasty as well as an extensor tendon repair will be necessary.

It is often recommended to use extensor carpi ulnaris tendon for the repair of the extensors to the little finger (plus the ring finger if that also has ruptured). If the wrist is fixed and hence not needing muscle control, this is acceptable. However, if the wrist is mobile and still used in its important ulnar deviating role, it is better not to use this tendon as a motor. If only the little-finger tendon is lost, since there is little normal separation of movement from that of the ring finger, the proximal end of the ruptured tendon may be attached proximally to the ring-finger tendon (**Figure a**, below).

If the ring-finger and little-finger tendons have ruptured they can be similarly anchored to the middle-finger tendon if that is intact (**Figure b**) but often in rheumatoid disease it is also damaged. Further damage will be prevented and repair will probably occur after synovectomy but it is risky to add too great a load. In any case there is much to be said for isolating the functions of the index and middle fingers from those of the ring and little fingers if at all possible, even in rheumatoid disease. Thus if the middle-finger tendon is ruptured it can be linked most satisfactorily to those of the index finger if they are in a satisfactory state, using another method for the ring and little fingers. Alternatively, the extensor indicis proprius can be diverted distally, passed through a slit in the divided tendons and then sutured to them individually under tension (**Figure c**). If all the finger tendons are ruptured in the presence of an intact extensor pollicis longus it is justifiable to divide this tendon distally and pass it through slits in the distal ends of the ruptured tendons and suture individually under tension. The extensor pollicis longus is then repaired with an extensor pollicis brevis transplant. If the extensor pollicis longus is also ruptured then it should be repaired by an extensor pollicis

brevis or abductor pollicis longus transplant and the fingers treated separately.

If all the tendons have ruptured recently and their own muscles are still in reasonable state, there is much to be said for attempting a more direct repair. An intramuscular tendon slide is excellent but may not appeal. If the proximal tendons are thick enough they may be split and the excised or reflected split used as bridge grafts; if not, one proximal tendon of a pair can be excised joining the two muscles to the remaining tendon and the excised piece used as a bridge graft to the joined distal tendons of the two fingers. Thus the index-finger and middle-finger tendons can be paired, as can the ring-finger and little-finger tendons.

If the extensor tendons are not suitable for effective tendon repair then all the metacarpophalangeal joints should be stabilized in extension using straight pegs, which will allow flexion and extension of the proximal interphalangeal and terminal interphalangeal joints to occur via the intrinsic muscles.

After rupture of the extensor tendons, the metacarpophalangeal joints should be kept in the extended position for 3–4 weeks in plaster of Paris, but the proximal interphalangeal should be allowed complete freedom of movement.

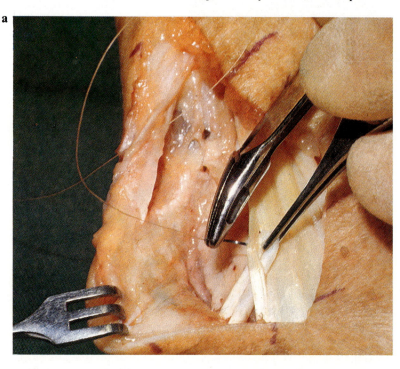

a The ruptured distal extensor tendon stump of the little finger is sutured to that of the ring finger. Care must be taken that at the suture the fingers must both be in extension and the ring-finger tendon as well as the stump taut. The proximal stump may also be sutured to the ring-finger tendon, thus keeping the little-finger muscle active.

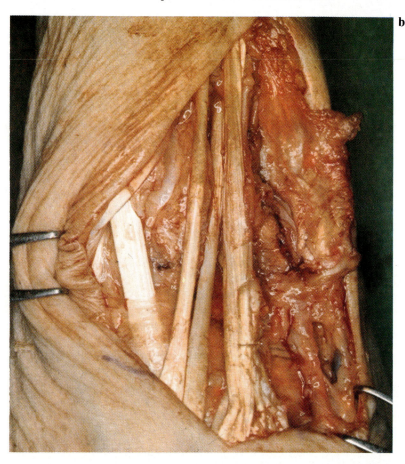

b Sometimes the ring-finger and little-finger tendons may be joined to the intact middle-finger tendon as in **Figure a** if other means cannot reasonably be used.

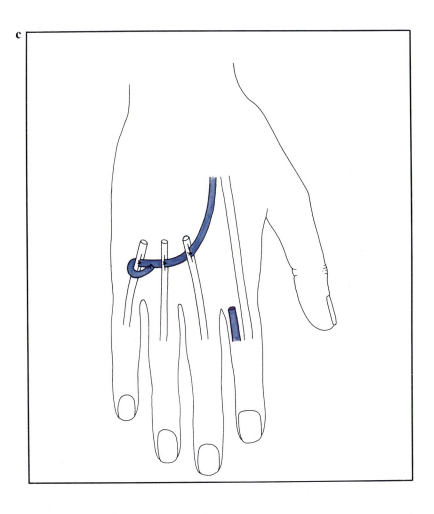

c In a long-standing rupture where other means cannot reasonably be used the extensor indicis proprius may be used as a common motor for middle-, ring- and little-finger extension.

Extensor digitorum tendon bridge graft

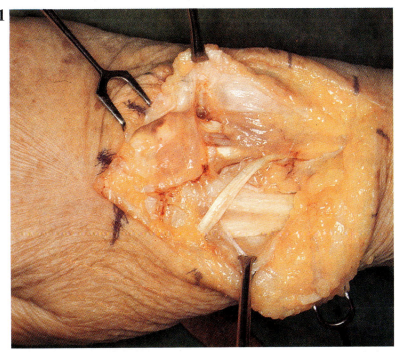

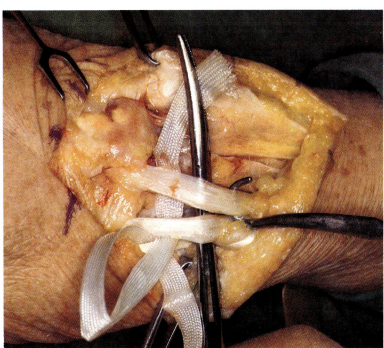

1 The hand is opened as for an extensor tenosynovectomy and the extensor expansion retracted. The extensor carpi radialis and extensor pollicis longus tendons have been cleared of synovium. The digital mass of synovium has been divided to show the tendons which are intact under the retinaculum.

2 The index-finger tendons have now been cleared and the intact cleared tendons are now collected together in tape for easy retraction.

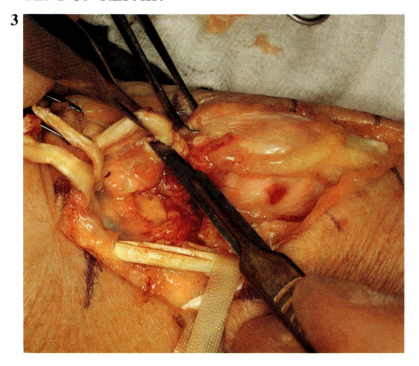

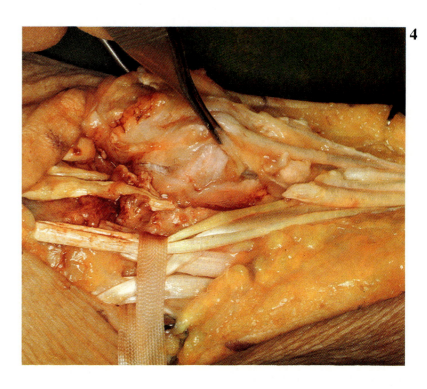

3 The distal ends of the tendon to the middle, ring and little fingers are now cleared.

4 Followed by the proximal ends. The distal radio-ulnar joint is heavily affected by the disease and requires synovectomy and removal of the distal end of the bone. Note, however, that the tendons have ruptured distal to the ulnar head (though the proximal ends have retracted by muscle contraction).

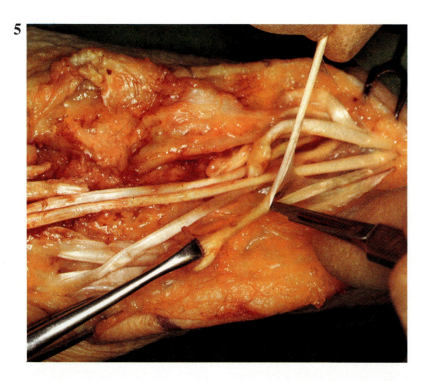

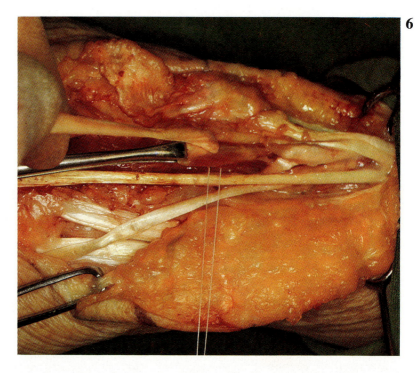

5 The proximal tendon to the middle finger has been partially divided close to the muscle and is being split, taking off half the thickness for use as a graft.

6 The last few millimetres of the tendon have been left intact and a suture passed through to hold this attachment. The trimmed end of the tendon will then be stitched into the graft to produce a neat union.

7

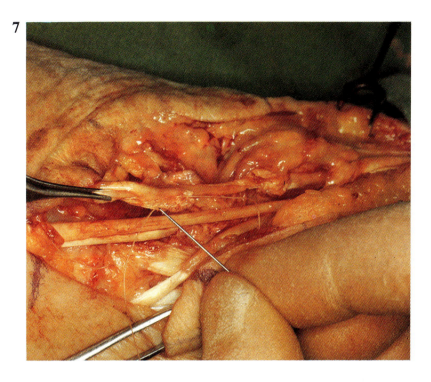

8

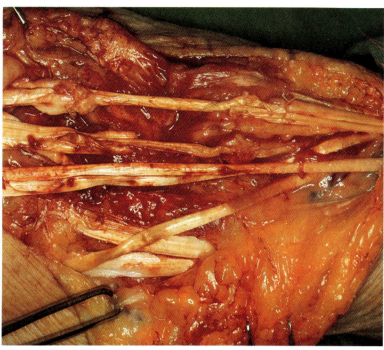

7 A button-hole is then made in the trimmed end of the distal tendon, the graft passed through and sutured using Dexon, Prolene or fine silk. The tendon ends are carefully sutured in to give a neat junction. Note that the graft is pulled through the button-hole so that there is gentle tension from the muscle with the finger in extension, and then fixed.

8 A similar bridge has been obtained from the existing tendons for the ring finger and little finger, the tendons joined together proximally and distally to the graft. There must be similar tension on all the fingers in extension.

9

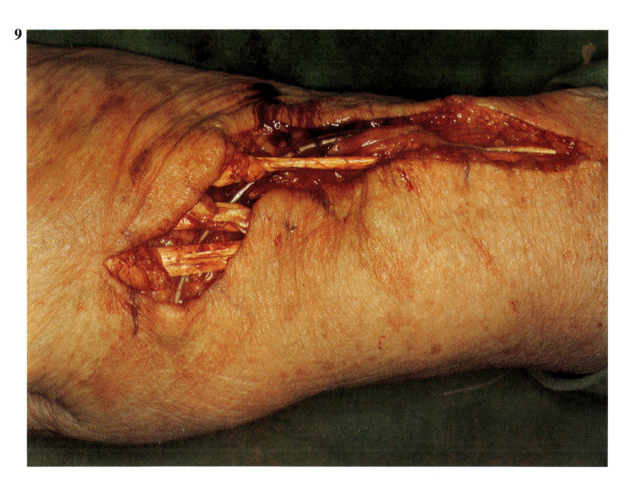

9 A suction drain has been inserted and the wound is ready for suture. As the proximal tendon sutures would be beneath the retinaculum this is not replaced over their surface.

Rupture of the long flexor tendon to the thumb

The flexor pollicis longus is the commonest flexor tendon to rupture in rheumatoid disease. The rupture can occur at three sites: (1) by avulsion from its insertion; (2) at the level of the metacarpophalangeal joint; and (3) in the carpal tunnel.

Three different methods of repair are advocated, depending on the site of rupture:

1 In avulsion, the repair is ideally by tendon graft.
2 At the level of the metacarpophalangeal joint, the repair can be made by using a tendon transplant, preferably the flexor sublimis of the ring finger, or by tendon graft if the flexor pollicis longus muscle is still in good working order.
3 Rupture in the carpal tunnel can be repaired by a bridge graft.

Whichever method is used, the first metacarpophalangeal joint should be stabilized with a straight peg or other method of arthrodesis at the same time as the tendon repair, if there is a flexion deformity, instability, or strong radiological evidence of destruction. If this is not done the joint will remain permanently flexed after immobilization in the flexed position in plaster of Paris, as will be needed for 3–4 weeks.

The method of tendon graft is shown and is essentially the same whether the rupture has occurred at the insertion (avulsion) or more proximally.

When the tendon is ruptured at the level of the metacarpophalangeal joint crease, an alternative to grafting is a tendon transplant. The flexor sublimis (superficialis) of the ring finger is exposed in the palm at the level of the proximal digital crease, and then divided. It is passed across the palm to the base of the thumb, where it enters a slit in the base of the distal end of the flexor pollicis, and is sutured under tension.

Where the flexor pollicis ruptures in the carpal tunnel, the thenar incision must be extended to open the carpal tunnel and expose the rupture. Once the tendon ends are identified, the gap between can be repaired by a bridge graft as in the finger (see page 145). Alternatively, half of the proximal end of the tendon is turned over on itself, to bridge the gap, and is sutured to the distal end (**Figure 7.1**, page 113) or an intramuscular slide of the tendon can be used.

Occasionally, a patient may present with a long-standing rupture of flexor pollicis longus where the muscle is atrophic and no longer suitable for graft. If the metacarpophalangeal joint functions well under control of the short muscles and a sublimis transfer is considered unreasonable, an excellent result can usually be achieved by arthrodesis of the interphalangeal joint in a suitable position, as described in Chapter 8.

Both flexor pollicis longus and the index-finger flexors may rupture together (this is less common in the other fingers). They can be treated together by grafts but if there are difficulties then, as for the thumb, interphalangeal arthrodesis may be performed as long as the metacarpophalangeal joint is in good mechanical control from the short muscles and is not seriously affected by disease.

Flexor pollicis longus tendon graft

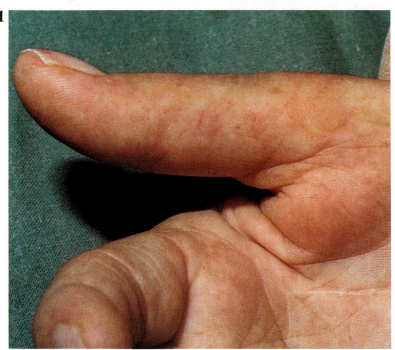

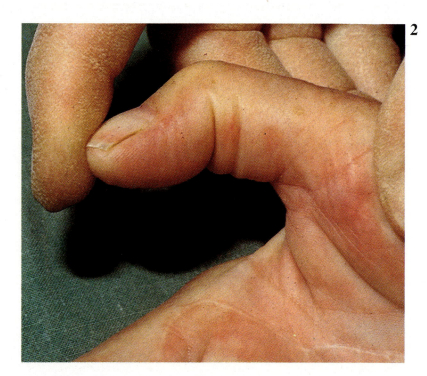

1 The thumb at rest, showing normal extension of the joint. Active flexion is not possible.

2 The passive range of 45° is demonstrated. If the joint is stiff there is little point in carrying out the operation.

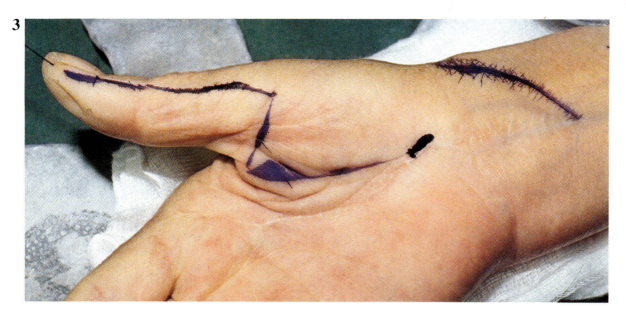

3 The incision passes along the radial side of the thumb, then crosses the proximal crease, and finally extends proximally in the thenar crease.

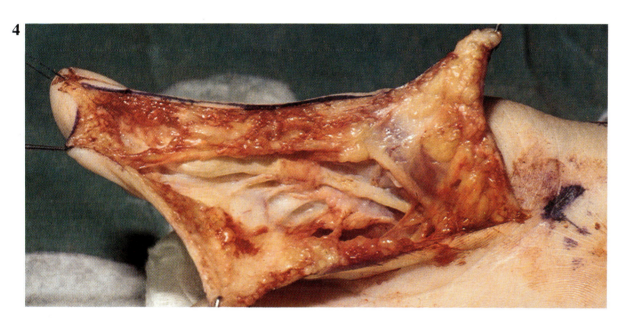

4 The radial digital nerve is exposed. Some fibrous reconstitution of the flexor tendon is visible.

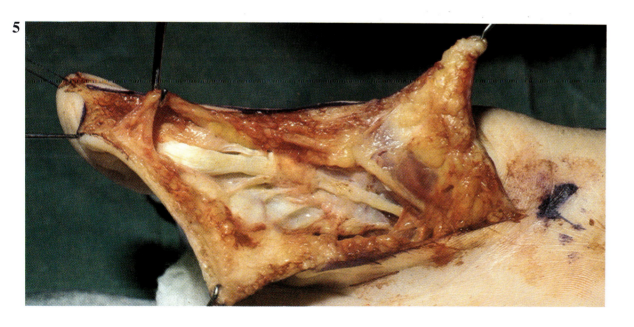

5 A pulley of the fibrous flexor sheath has been left over the proximal phalanx. The distal part of the flexor tendon can be seen, and proximal to the pulley the reconstituted tendon of fibrous tissue. The false tendon is removed, and the distal divided section is dissected distally to its attachment, onto the terminal phalanx.

6

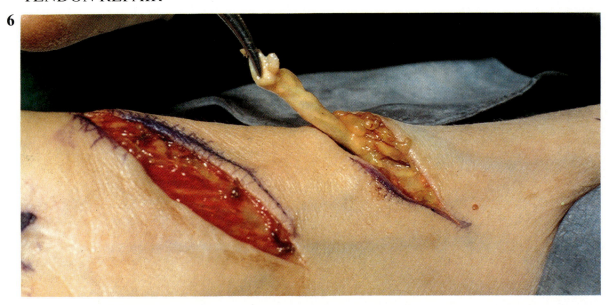

6 The proximal ruptured end of the flexor pollicis longus is found in the forearm, and held in forceps. Note the distorted character of the tendon bundles at the site of rupture.

7

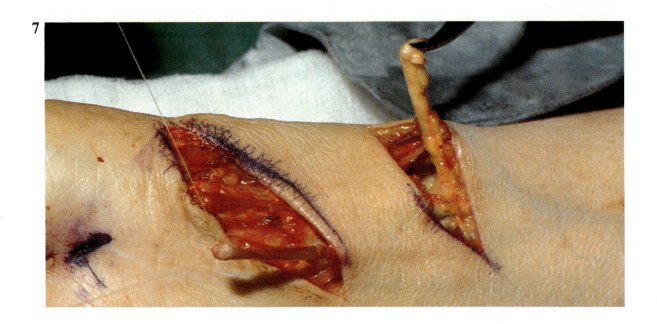

7 Through an oblique incision at the wrist crease, the tendon of the palmaris longus is defined, a stitch is inserted and the tendon divided.

8

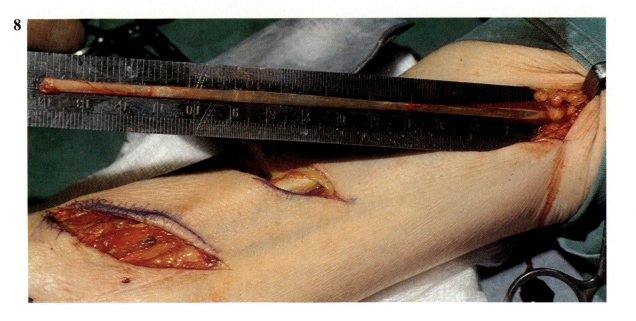

8 The palmaris tendon is dissected proximally through oblique incisions, until 14–17 cm can be measured on the ruler. A suture is now passed through the proximal end and the tendon divided. It is advisable to take the full 17 cm if available but here only 14 cm was possible.

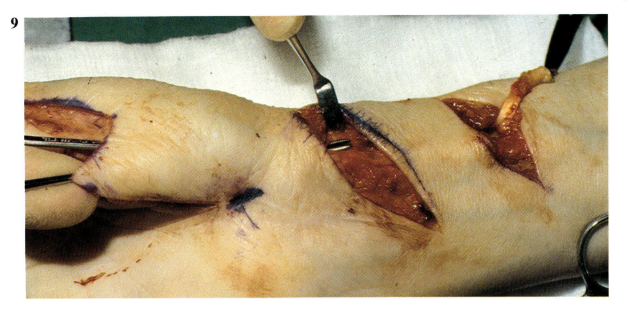

9 An artery clip is passed proximally from the palmar exposure and presents in the wound at the wrist, where it takes hold of the stitch on the distal end of the tendon graft. The graft must not be held directly with forceps or it will be damaged.

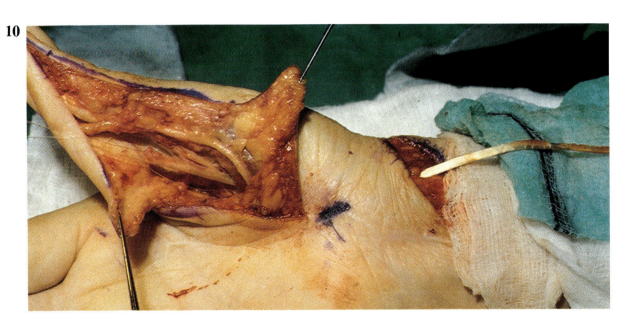

10 The tendon graft is pulled through into the palm.

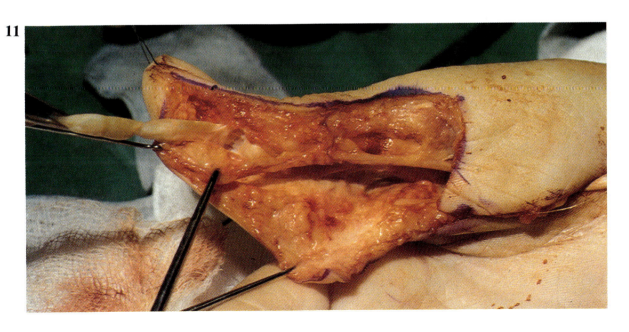

11 The distal end of the flexor tendon is retracted distally and excised, leaving a small stump for suture to the tendon graft. The bone in this area is scarified to facilitate adhesions forming with the tendon graft.

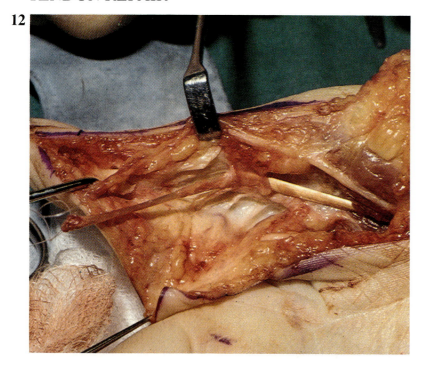

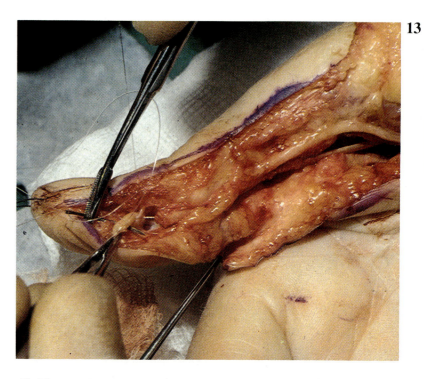

12 The tendon graft has been passed beneath the pulley, and the sutures at the terminal end are threaded onto two small, curved, cutting needles, which are then passed through the distal stump of the flexor tendon. Again tendon ends must not be gripped by forceps.

13 The needles are then doubled back through the tendon, so that the graft can be drawn up beneath the distal tendon stump. This makes a very secure junction, well beyond the level of the volar plate.

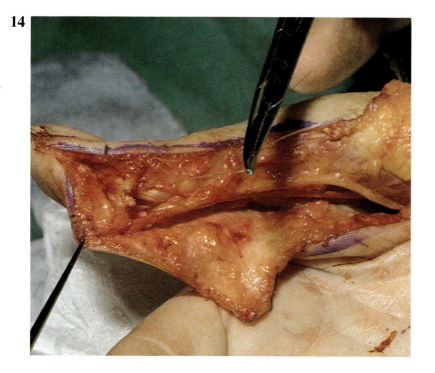

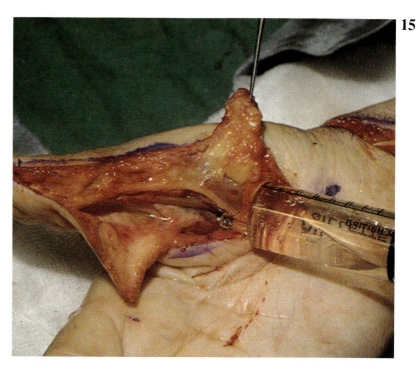

14 The final suture is made.

15 An antibiotic solution is inserted into the wound.

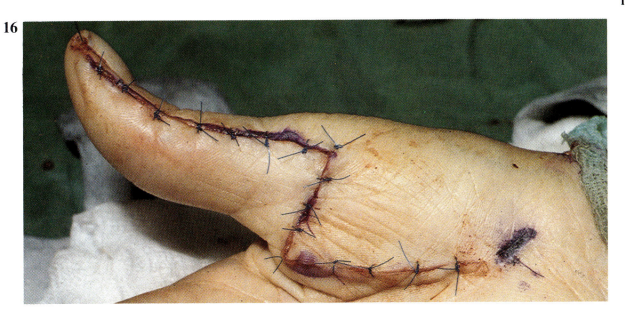

16 The thumb wound is closed.

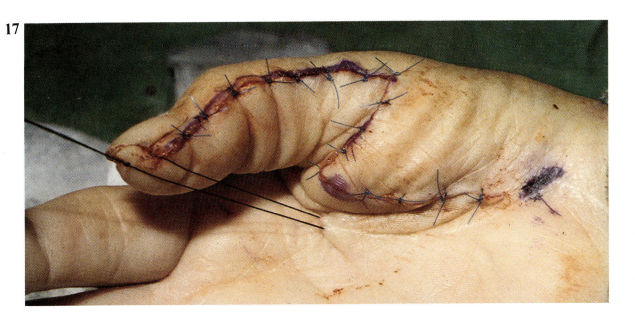

17 The tip of the thumb is sutured to the palm to prevent an accidental extension injury after the proximal suture has been made, and during the period of dressing and plaster fixation.

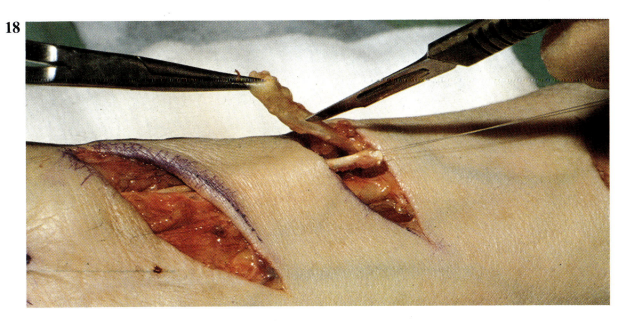

18 The distal end of the flexor tendon in the forearm is split with a knife.

19

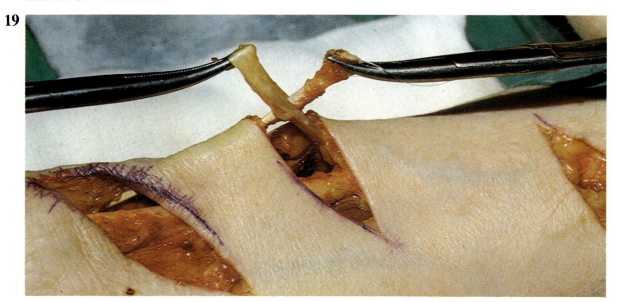

19 The proximal end of the tendon graft is passed through the slit in the flexor tendon, as in the button-hole technique. Tension is exerted on the graft; any surplus will be removed later.

20

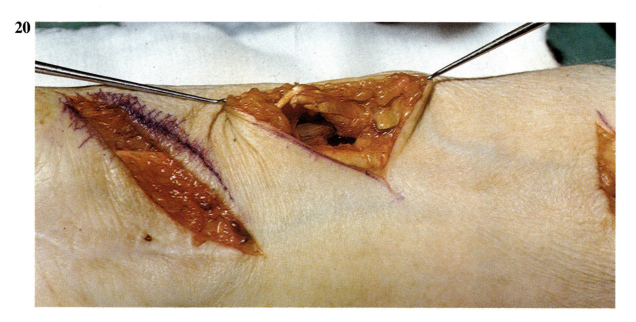

20 The junction is secured with white braided nylon sutures, the surplus tendon carefully sutured to give a neat surface and any surplus material trimmed off.

21

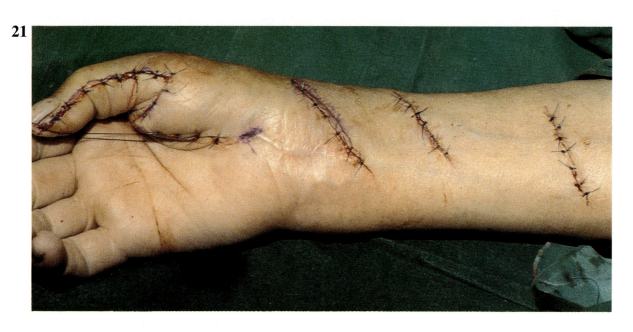

21 All wounds were closed after removal of the tourniquet and bleeding fully controlled.

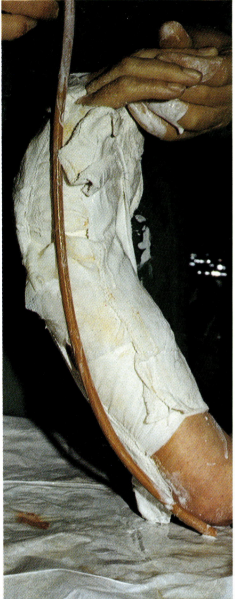 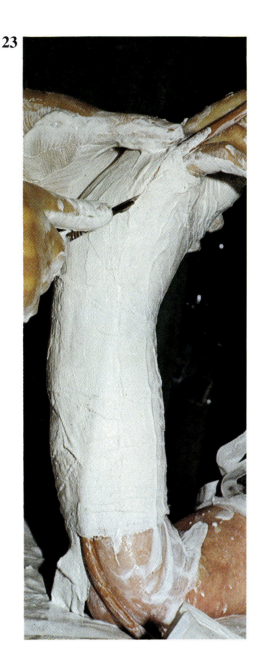 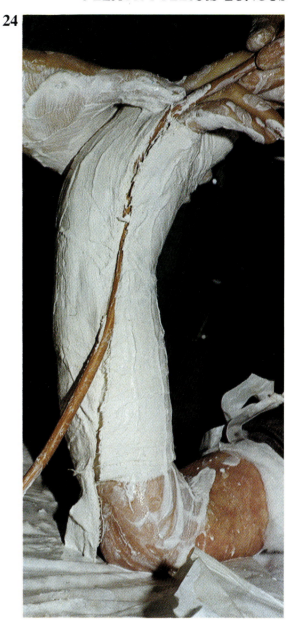

22 A plaster of Paris splint is applied incorporating a rubber tube. The wrist is in 25–30° of flexion, and the terminal joint of the thumb is plastered in flexion.

23 The plaster of Paris splint is split over the rubber tube to avoid damaging the skin.

24 The tube is removed and a wet cotton bandage is applied. It is advisable to split the plaster, because if severe postoperative swelling should occur then opening the plaster is a simple procedure. The hand and arm should be elevated for 4 or 5 days. The patient should then wear a sling, and exercise the shoulder and elbow in elevation. Three and a half weeks later, the plaster of Paris and sutures were removed. The end-result showed good scars with full thumb extension and 35° active flexion at the interphalangeal joint, providing a stable precision pinch.

Digital flexor tendon rupture

Rupture can occur to either or both of the flexor tendons of the fingers, the most commonly affected being those of the index and middle fingers. Hence, when it occurs, some form of treatment is essential. The most common sites of rupture are at the distal end of the carpal tunnel, and at the entrance to the fibrous flexor sheath of the fingers, but rupture within the fibrous sheath is by no means uncommon. Thus ruptures when they occur are often distal to the attachment of the lumbrical muscle to the profundus tendon and in the so-called 'no-man's

land' of tendon repair. However, as there will inevitably be loss of a length of necrotic tendon there is no question of end-to-end anastomosis and hence a tendon graft is the treatment of choice. Within this region the graft must be a thin tendon to allow for the swelling that will inevitably occur in the graft. Hence the choice is palmaris longus (when present), as shown, or one of the short toe extensor tendons; plantaris is usable but tends to be too thick. More proximally the thickness of the graft is less important. —Continued on page 140

Flexor tendon graft to the index finger

1

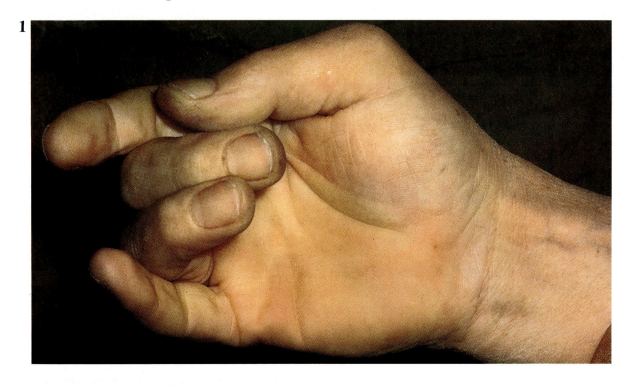

1 Loss of flexion in the index finger makes pinch between it and the thumb impossible. This can be a serious disability and also any straight finger gets in the way. Repair of function is therefore necessary. The 'empty' feel in the finger indicates that rupture has occurred there rather than more proximally.

2

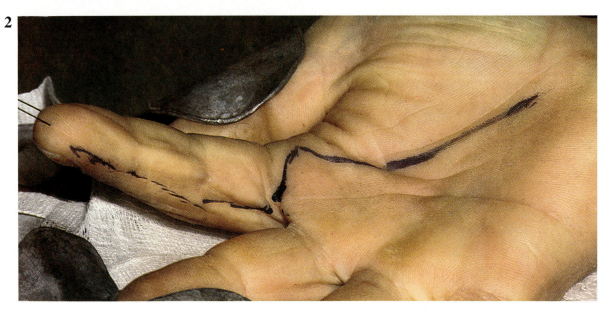

2 The line of incision is made along the ulnar side of the index finger. Damage to the digital nerves which are vital for sensation, must be avoided.

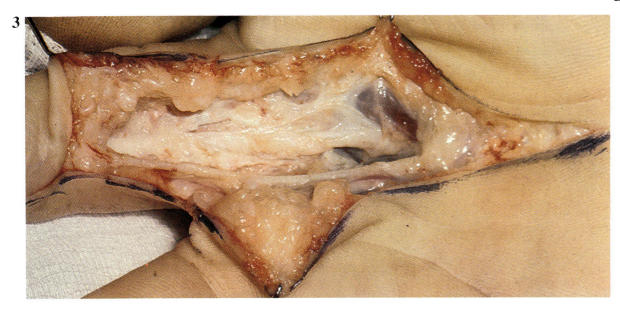

3 The ulnar digital nerve is exposed, but there is no visible flexor tendon. There has been an attempt to reconstitute the tendon with scar tissue.

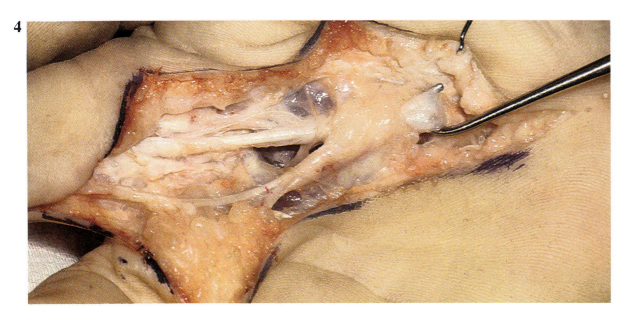

4 The sublimis tendon has been exposed, and is held in a blunt hook. The attempt to reconstitute this tendon is clearly defined distally.

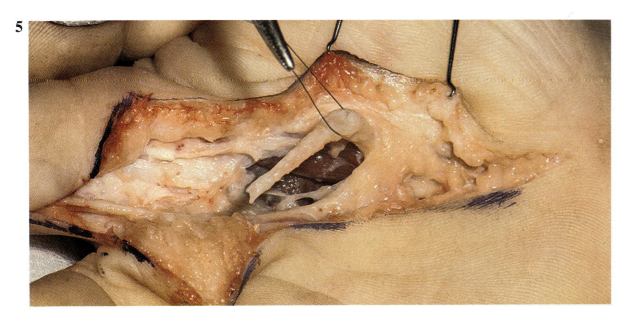

5 The flexor sublimis tendon is held with a traction stitch and the tendon subsequently removed.

135

6

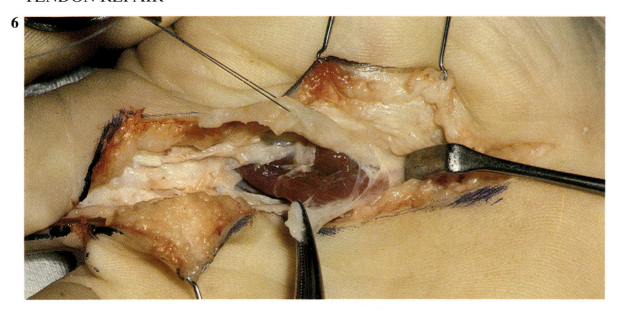

6 The profundus tendon is identified and its ruptured end held with an artery clip. The attachment of the lumbrical muscle to the tendon can be seen and this has prevented the tendon being pulled more proximally.

7

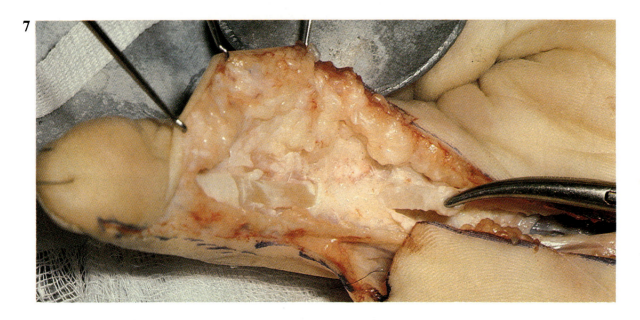

7 The fibrous flexor sheath is opened distally and pulleys of sheath are left over the proximal and middle phalanges. It is essential to retain these pulleys. If for any reason they are lost or too stretched owing to synovial bulk, as sometimes occurs in rheumatoid disease, they must be reconstituted otherwise the tendon will 'bow string' and digital flexion will be ineffective.

8

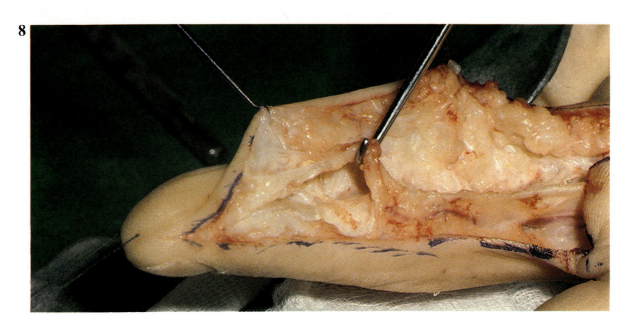

8 The neuro-vascular bundle is retracted anteriorly, to allow access to the terminal phalanx.

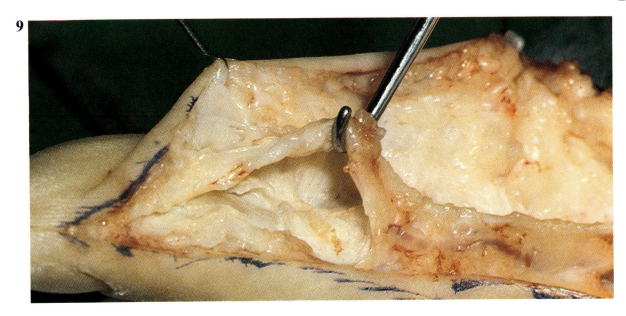

9 As the bundle is held anteriorly the volar plate of the terminal interphalangeal joint can be seen.

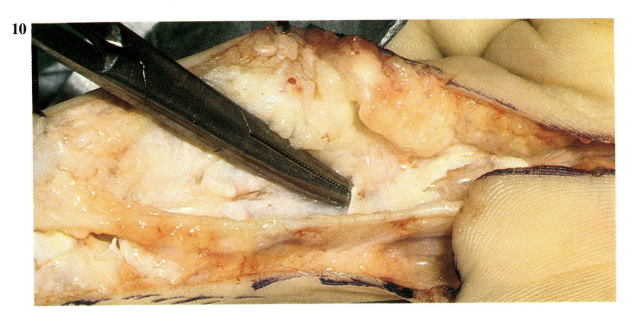

10 The proximal pulley is cleared of any adhesions by the insertion of an artery clip beneath it.

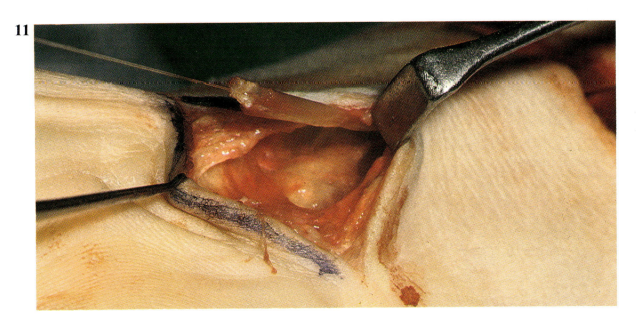

11 The palmaris longus tendon is exposed in the forearm through transverse incision as for the flexor pollicis longus graft. The divided distal end is held on a figure-of-eight stitch, using 4/0 white nylon suture. If, as commonly occurs, there is no palmaris longus a short extensor tendon of a toe may be used or failing that plantaris; but plantaris is usually too thick and with the severe swelling which occurs in the graft often becomes' adherent within the finger.

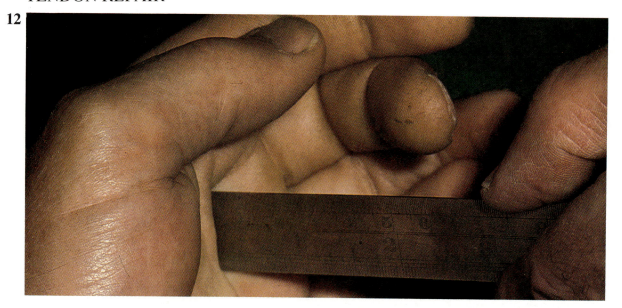

12 A measurement is made on the normal hand of the distance from the tip of the index finger to the palm. This gives an indication of the length of the flexor tendon which is to be replaced in the damaged hand by an estimation of tension (SHH).

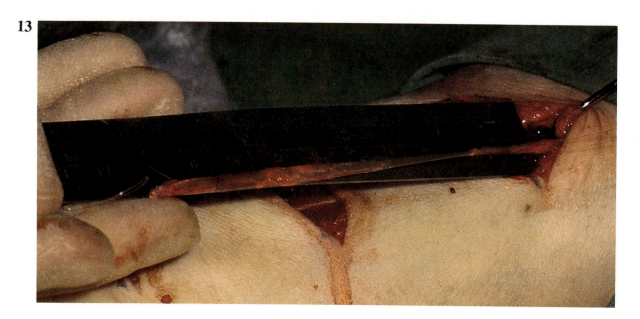

13 The length of tendon graft to be removed is measured. The index finger usually requires 9–9.5 cm (SHH).

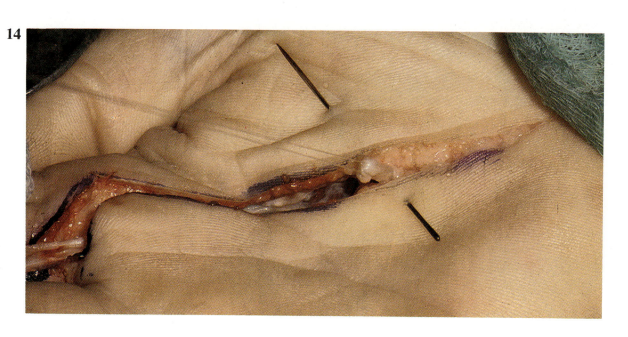

14 The proximal end of the cut flexor tendon is transfixed with a straight needle to prevent retraction. The tendon end is held on a figure-of-eight stitch, in which both ends finish in the terminal part of the tendon. See **Figure 19a**, page 140.

15

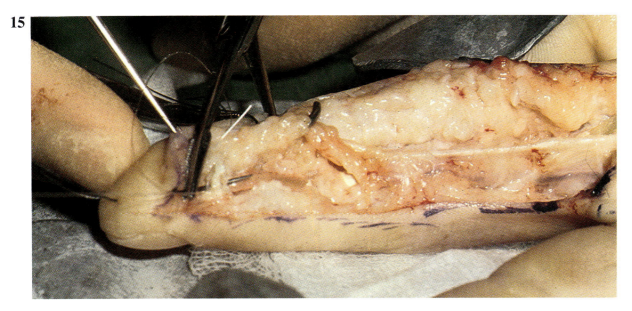

15 The tendon graft is passed beneath the pulley over the proximal phalanx, and then beneath that over the middle phalanx. The proximal pulley is about 1 cm wide and that over the middle phalanx 0.5 cm. Needles are attached to both ends of the suture in the tendon graft, and both are passed through the distal end of the ruptured tendon, then doubled back through the distal end, and tied, so that the tendon graft is tucked under the trimmed distal stump of the flexor profundus. The underlying bone has been scarified to encourage adhesions to the tendon graft.

16

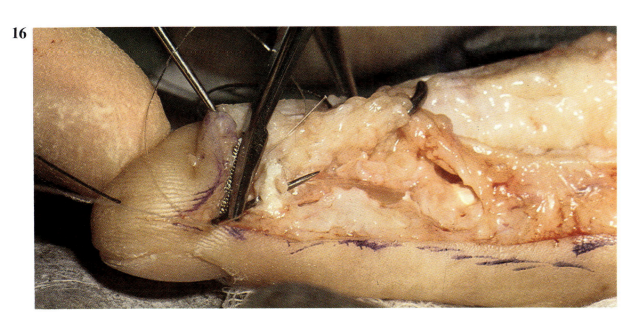

16 The stitch can be seen being doubled back through the distal stump of the flexor profundus tendon.

17

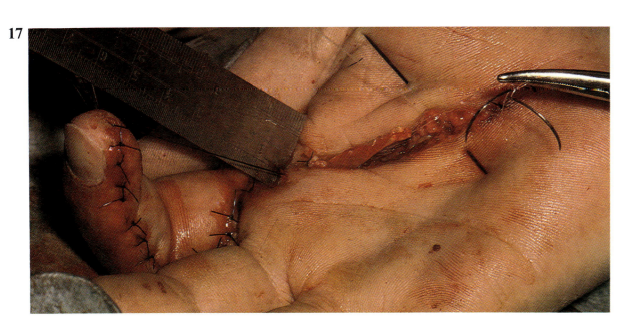

17 The fingertip is sutured to the palm, at the same position as the normal index finger on the opposite hand. The incision in the finger is then closed and, after removal of the excess tendon graft, the proximal suture is established by a double figure-of-eight suture, so that the knots lie between the tendon ends (**Figure 19a**, page 140).

18

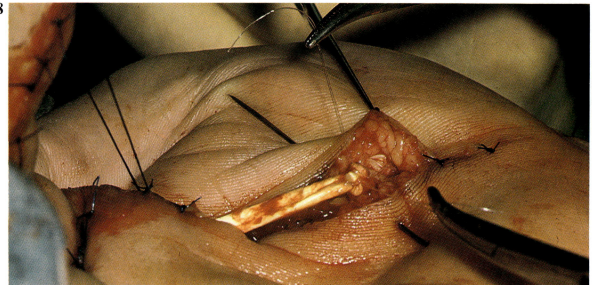

18 The proximal junction has been made, and the tendon graft can be seen neatly sutured to the proximal stump of profundus. The straight needle which has been stabilizing the proximal part of the flexor profundus is then removed. At this point the tourniquet is released and bleeding points secured before the wound is repaired. A plaster of Paris splint is applied and is split over a rubber tube as for a flexor pollicis longus graft. After 3 weeks, intensive exercises are encouraged, for 10–15 minutes every hour. The patient is advised before the operation that recovery of movements can be achieved only by his own efforts.

19 a

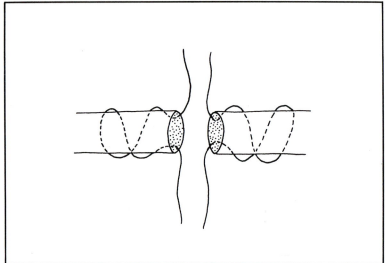

b

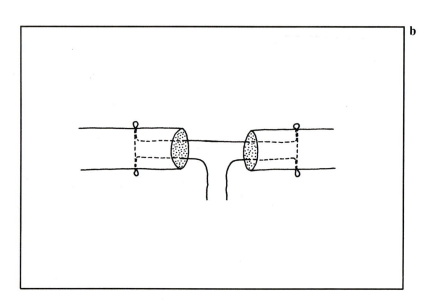

19a A diagram of the figure-of-eight method of end-to-end suture used in this operation. The 2 knots are thus buried between the tendon ends.

19b Another commonly used method. Note that if skin-hooks are put under the loops the joining strand can be pulled tight. The process is thus repeated on the loops of the free ends and these ends pulled up and tied.

—Continued from page 134

In rheumatoid disease it is often proper to carry out procedures which would not be acceptable in 'clean' traumatic cases.

If profundus is ruptured in 'no-man's-land' the proper practice may be to graft profundus and to excise sublimis in whole or part or to leave enough over the proximal inter-phalangeal joint as a tenodesis to prevent swan's-neck deformity. Such would be the ideal in rheumatoid disease but where profundus ruptures after an initial synovectomy, leaving a good sublimis tendon intact, it is often reasonable to limit further damage by leaving sublimis to control the proximal interphalangeal joint and to connect the terminal joint in slight flexion by arthrodesis.

Sublimis graft for a profundus tendon

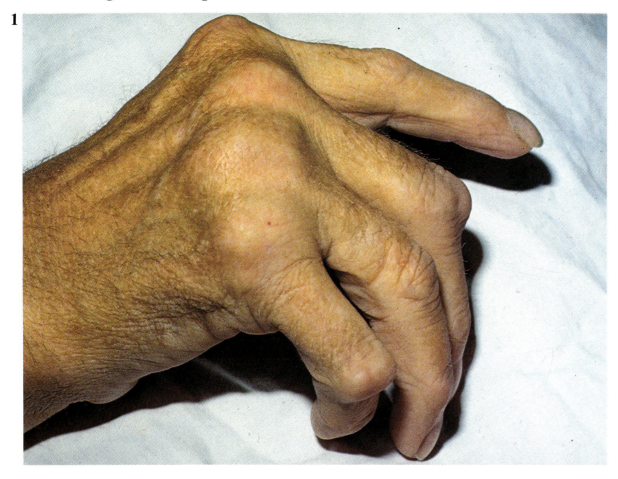

1 The patient had a clinically obvious rupture of both the flexor tendons to the index finger together with marked tenosynovial thickening in the palm.

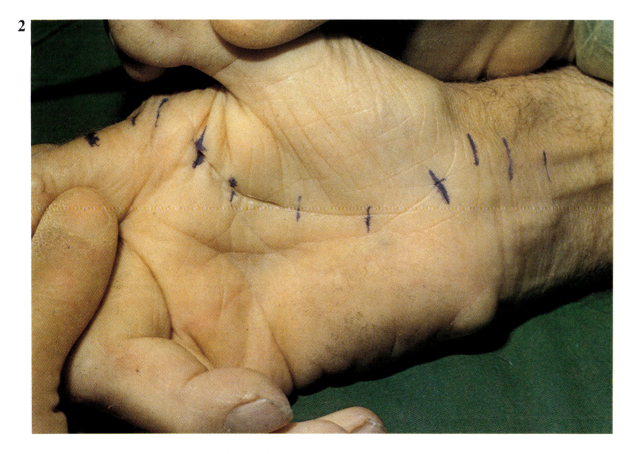

2 The hand is marked up as for a proximal flexor synovectomy but with the option to continue up the finger if necessary. It was expected from the bulk over the proximal phalanx of the finger that the tendons were intact here and that the rupture was likely to be in the palm.

3

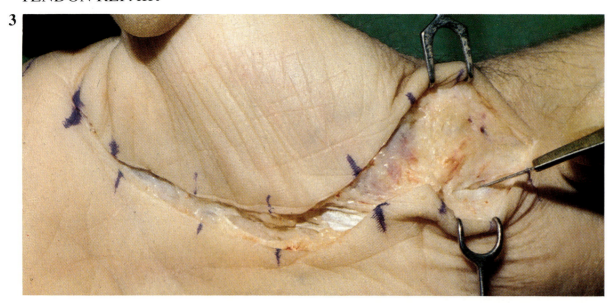

3 The incision proceeds, taking care to preserve the palmar branch of the median nerve at the heel of the hand.

4

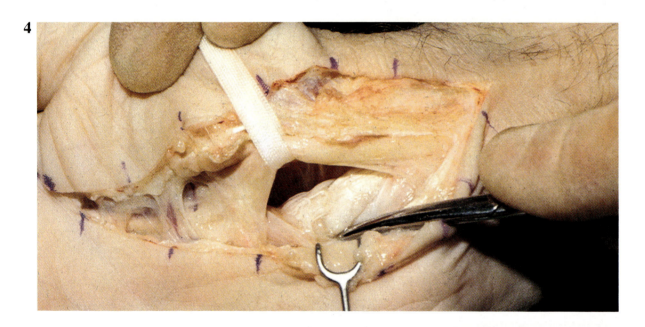

4 The median nerve is isolated from the matted mass of tendons and synovium in the palm and pulled clear by tape.

5

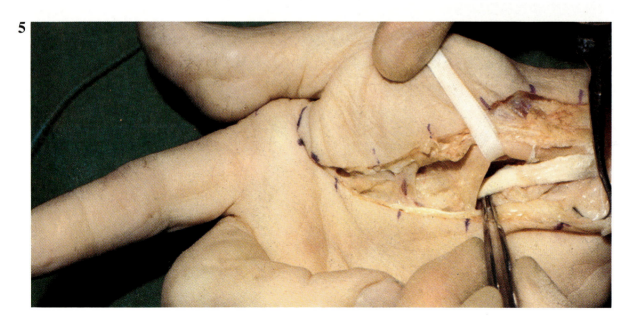

5 A systematic tenosynovectomy is then carried out proximally along the intact tendons.

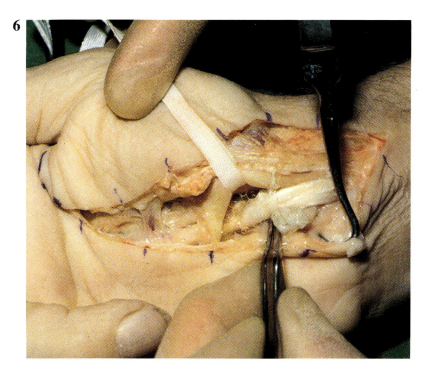

6 The sublimis (superficialis tendon) to the middle finger has intact fibres anteriorly but there is a mass of necrotic, ruptured fibres on the deep side with the deeper structures. The index-finger tendon is missing. Much serous fluid is seen in the depths of the wound.

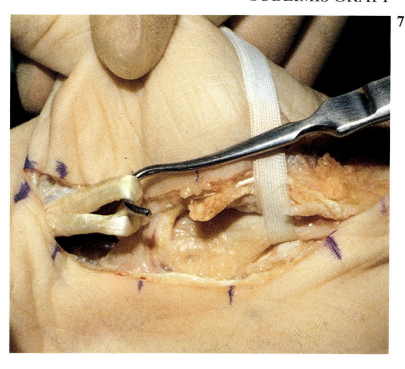

7 The affected tendons are found distally, shown to be intact and cleared of synovium.

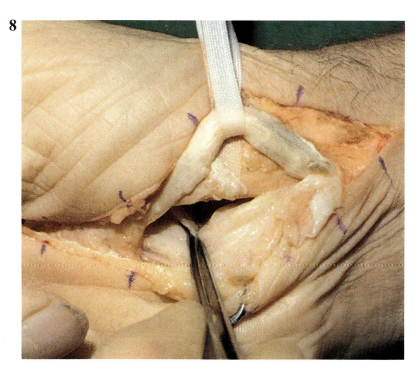

8 Attention is now turned to the mass of material containing the profundus tendons and the index sublimis.

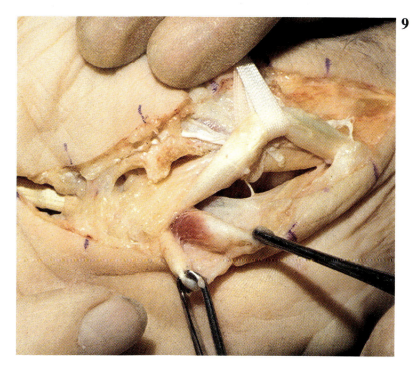

9 By clearing from distal to proximal along the index profundus tendon, the distal ruptured end is found close to the origin of the lumbrical muscle.

10

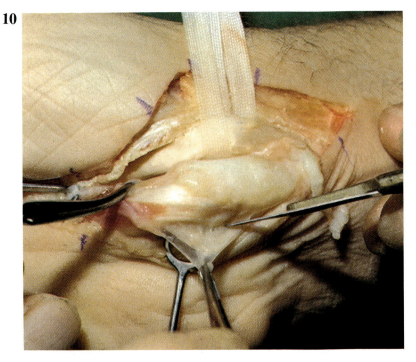

10 The remainder of the tendons are now cleared.

11

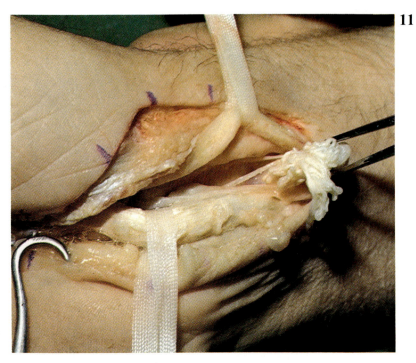

11 The proximal shredded end of sublimis is found together with necrotic shredded mass of the index profundus tendon.

12

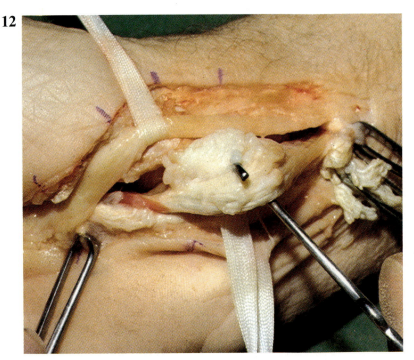

12 The two index-finger tendons' tips have been collected on Allis forceps whilst the remaining profundus tendons are cleaned. Both the middle-finger and ring-finger tendons show much necrotic material and swollen collagen, but after synovectomy should heal adequately.

13

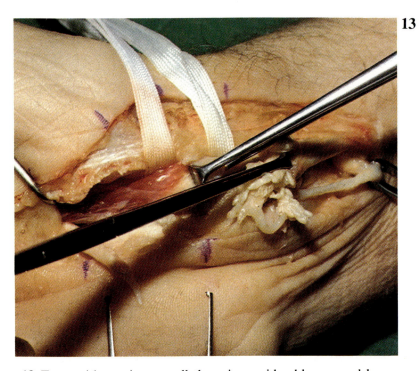

13 Even with maximum pull there is considerable gap and hence some form of bridge will be needed.

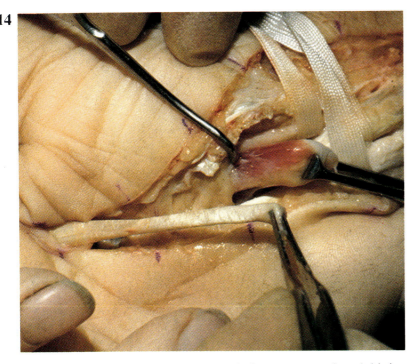

14 The sublimis tendon appears suitable for use as a graft and this is divided in the distal part of the palm and its stump sutured to the profundus tendon.

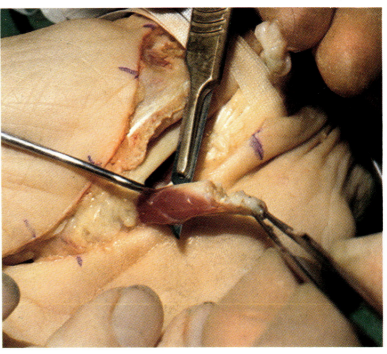

15 The ends of the profundus tendon have been cleared of necrotic material and a button-hole is being made for passage of the graft tendon.

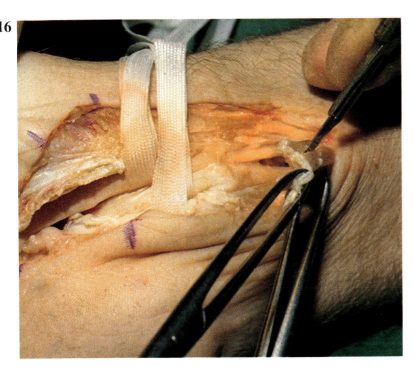

16 The proximal end is being treated likewise, the proximal end of sublimis having been sutured to it to give extra power.

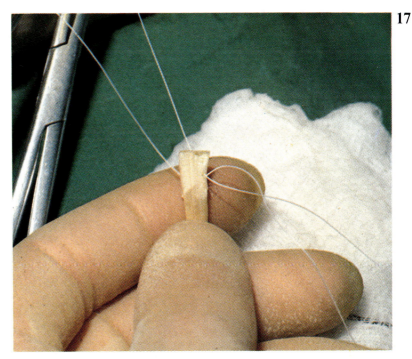

17 A suture has been passed through the graft and then each end of the suture is taken obliquely to leave the cut end of tendon.

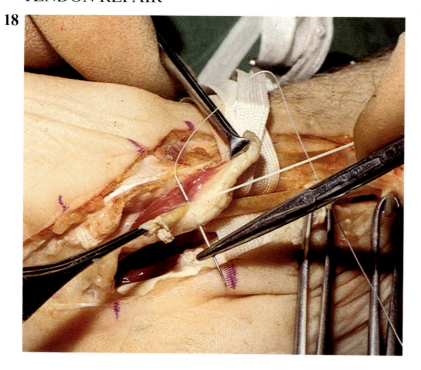

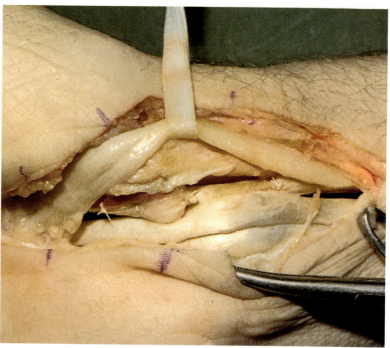

18 One end of the graft has been sutured to the proximal profundus tendon. The other end is now threaded through the button-hole in the distal stump. It will be adjusted to tension with the index finger pulled into the palm and a suture transfixing the tendons at the button-hole.

19 The two junctions have been sutured with neat joints.

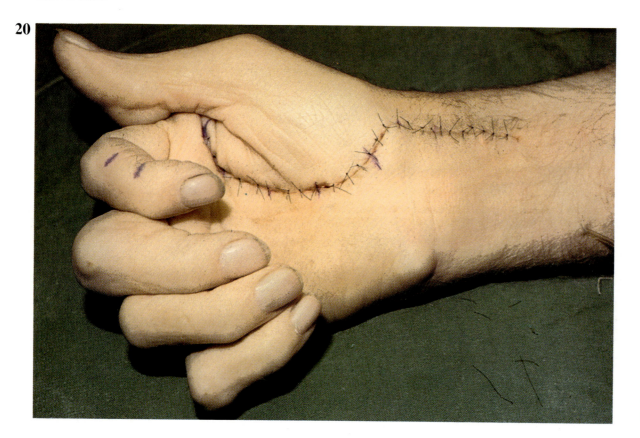

20 The wound has been sutured and the degree of tension on the index finger holds its tip into the palm. A suction drain is in place.

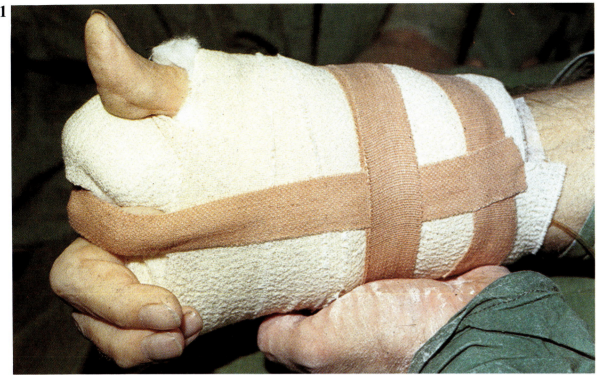

21 The hand is bandaged with controlling tape over the affected finger to prevent any risk of it being caught and its sutures disrupted.

More proximally, although a graft from external sources as for 'no-man's-land' may be ideal there may be need for the graft in the future and so sometimes less ideal methods are practised. As profundus is a more important muscle than sublimis, where both are ruptured a bridge graft may be taken from sublimis to repair profundus. If sublimis is intact and profundus ruptured a simple suture of profundus to sublimis with accurate tension will give good results, albeit with 'mass action'.

Rupture of profundus in the palm with an intact but damaged sublimis

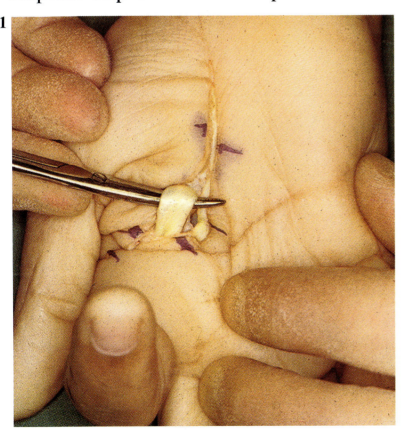

1 The findings of clinical examination suggested that the rupture was in the palm and not in the finger. An exploratory incision is therefore made in the distal part of the thenar crease which could be extended either or both ways as required. Both the tendons are found to be intact from here distally.

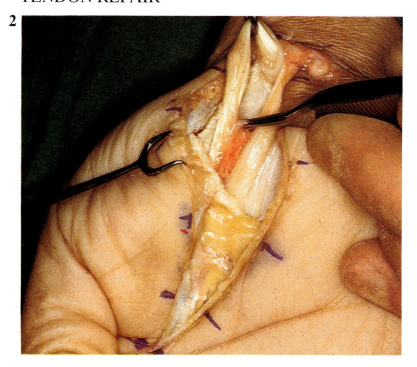

2 The incision is therefore carried proximally as far as for a flexor synovectomy which would need to be carried out at the same time as the repair. The index sublimis tendon has been found and cleared, showing only a tendon granuloma which, it was considered, would heal after synovectomy.

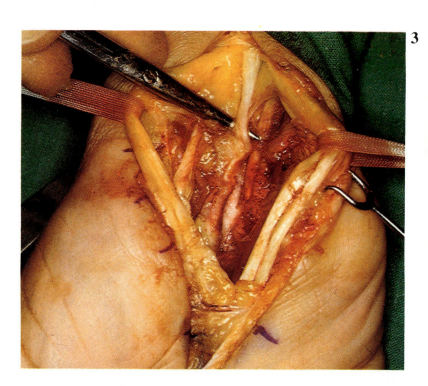

3 The synovectomy proceeds systematically. The proximal end of the profundus tendon has now been found in the carpal tunnel surrounded by a mass of highly vascular, active synovium. Unlike the previous case a cord of peritendinous material extended distally into the synovial mass to the distal tendon end.

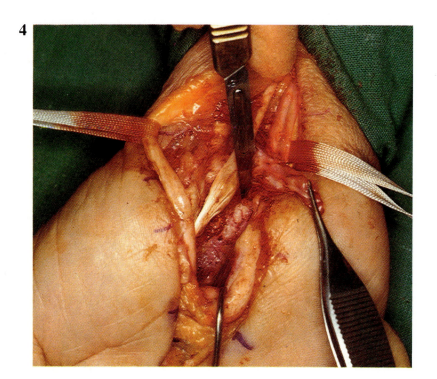

4 The vascular synovium is now cleared distally, following the peritendinous cord.

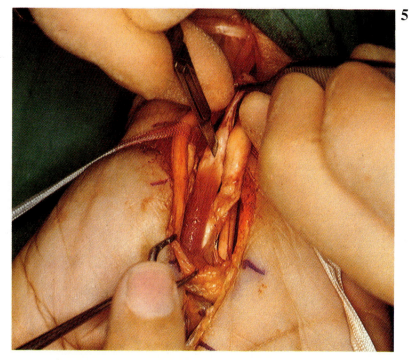

5 The distal end of the ruptured tendon is now identified and cleared, but leaving the cord linking the ruptured ends intact. As the sublimis tendon was damaged but intact, it was decided not to use it as a bridge graft but to link the profundus tendon to it. A split is being made in the distal profundus tendon.

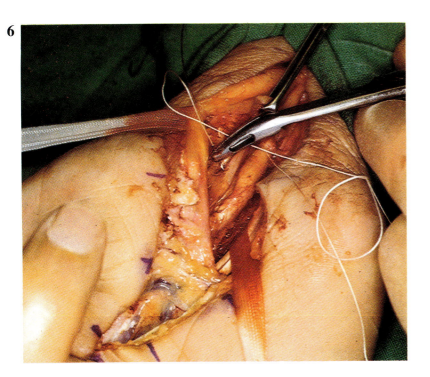

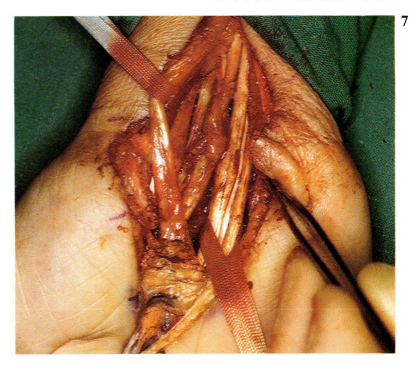

6 The split tendon is now sutured around the sublimis with the finger in flexion.

7 The proximal profundus tendon has been treated likewise, having been pulled distally. The bridge of peritendinous material between the profundus ends has been retained and is used folded to cover and support the granulomatous portion of sublimis, to which surface it has been sutured.

Fibrosing tenosynovitis

In the healing phases of the disease, tendon adhesions may occur which simulate ruptured tendon. Even with someone thoroughly versed in the treatment of rheumatoid disease and aware of this problem, misdiagnosis may occur. One such case is illustrated where a tendon rupture of flexor pollicis longus was diagnosed in the carpal tunnel. Usually the condition occurs in juvenile disease but it may follow very active flare-up in adult rheumatoid disease; the hand is rested during the active phase and then movement is found to be impossible, and the natural assumption is that the tendon has ruptured.

Fibrosing synovitis of the flexor pollicis longus tendon

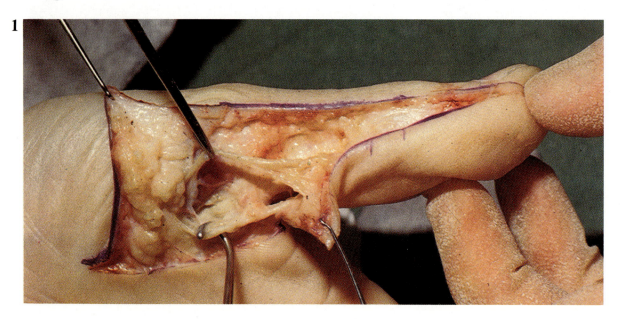

1 The incision for exposure of the long flexor tendon was carried out as described for tendon rupture, avoiding damage to the digital nerves and exposing the tendon in its sheath. Both digital nerves are retracted, and the dissection carried proximally separating the abductor and flexor pollicis brevis muscles.

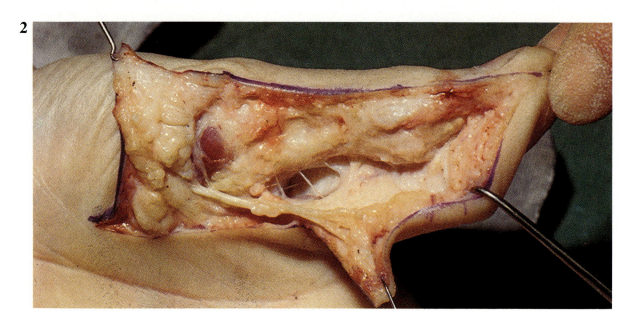

2 With the nerves dissected clear within the area exposed, the flexor tendon is inspected, revealing a thickened sheath and adhesions to the surrounding tissues.

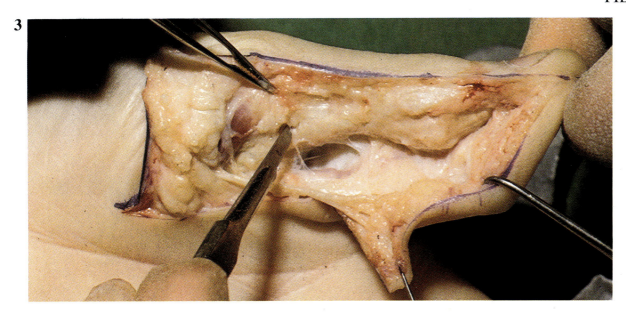

3 The sheath is excised, leaving a 1 cm wide pulley over the base of the proximal phalanx.

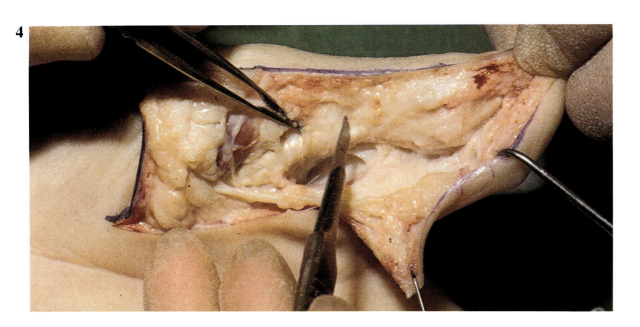

4 The distal part of the sheath is excised.

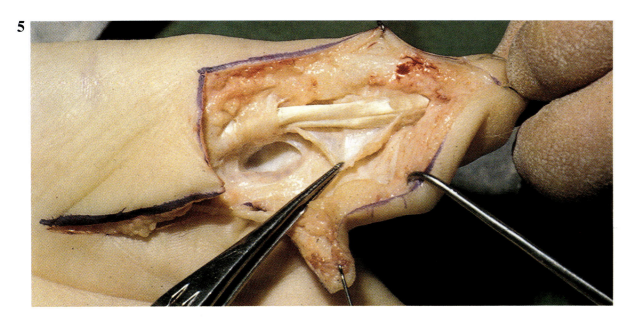

5 This revealed a tendon which was in continuity but lacked mobility.

6

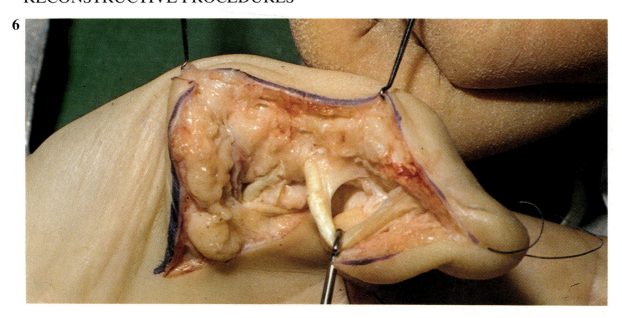

6 Dense adhesions can be seen passing from the tendon to the sheath overlying the bone.

7

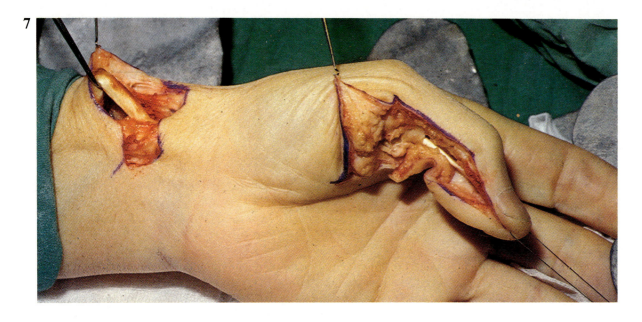

7 The proximal end of the long flexor tendon was exposed in the forearm, and after removal of adhesions, proximally and distally. it was possible to re-establish a freely gliding tendon, capable of flexing the terminal phalanx from 0 to 45°. The wound was closed after removal of the tourniquet. The hand was elevated and immediate active exercises started as soon as the patient had recovered from the anaesthetic.

This case demonstrates the healing stage of rheumatoid arthritis, in which synovial proliferation is converted into the stage of fibrosing synovitis. This can be disabling and in this case caused complete loss of flexion of the terminal joint of the thumb, simulating a cut flexor tendon.

8: Reconstructive and salvage procedures: arthrodesis, arthroplasty and various soft-tissue procedures

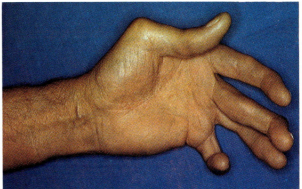

Rheumatoid and other arthropathies destroy joints. Joint replacement should be considered as a means of restoring active movement. The hand must always be regarded as a chain of joints which is only effective if the finely balanced control system is operational. In most arthropathies of the hand, particularly rheumatoid or psoriatic, extensive damage to the soft tissue seriously affects the control mechanism. Consequently, the replacement of damaged joints by mobile prostheses may be ineffective because of deficient mechanical control. It is therefore advisable to limit mobility to certain essential components and to fix other joints enabling control to be concentrated on essential mobile units. Although arthrodesis destroys the joint it often restores function to an essentially useless hand.

Most of the soft-tissue damage involves stretching of expansions or ligaments, and it might seem that simple reorganization of the stretched tissues would give good results. Stretching, however, leads to changes in the collagen and, no matter how competently the repair is performed, stretching is likely to continue unless new collagenous material is brought into the region.

The metacarpophalangeal joints are of prime functional importance to the fingers whereas the interphalangeal joints can often be fixed effectively in a semiflexed position. The metacarpophalangeal and particularly the interphalangeal joints of the thumb can be discarded provided that the carpometacarpal joint is effective. If the metacarpophalangeal joint of the thumb is good and well controlled by its muscles, it can assume the function of a lost carpometacarpal joint.

The thumb

Stabilization of a terminal joint

The terminal joint of the thumb is the one most likely to require arthrodesis. The terminal-interphalangeal digital joints are most commonly affected by degenerative arthritis (osteoarthrosis) or psoriatic arthropathy. Psoriatic arthropathy is a destructive joint disease and is often a source of instability which may become extreme at the terminal joints. If, however, the joints become fixed in unacceptable positions, the converse applies. Besides the digital joints, the terminal joint of the thumb may also be involved in both adult and juvenile rheumatoid disease. Hyperextension of the interphalangeal thumb joint may lead to loss of flexion or avulsion of the flexor tendon with ultimate instability.

This may be secondary to deformity at the metacarpophalangeal thumb joint, as in the 'Z-deformity', in which a flexion deformity occurs at the metacarpophalangeal joint with a secondary hyperextension at the interphalangeal joint (**Figure 8.1**). These secondary changes at the terminal joint can usually be avoided by early correction of the flexion deformity at the metacarpophalangeal joint, usually by arthrodesis.

As an alternative to tendon repair in cases of rupture of the flexor pollicis longus tendon, the thumb interphalangeal joint can profitably be fixed if the short muscles give effective control of the metacarpophalangeal joint.

Lateral instability of the thumb interphalangeal joint is common due to gross joint destruction in both psoriatic arthropathy and in juvenile and adult rheumatoid arthritis. Consequently the patient is severely disabled; a stable pinch becomes impossible and all effective precision action between thumb and fingers is lost. This situation occurs particularly in patients in whom pad-to-pad pinch has been replaced by lateral pinch due to other deformities of the hand.

It is common practice to cut out the joint when fixing a digital joint, thus enabling correct angulation of the bone ends for accurate apposition; this is then fixed by cross Kirschner wires. However, the technique appears much easier than it is in practice. The effort required to drill the wire obliquely through the bone cortex sometimes leads to a change in direction so that accurate replacement of the wire is not always easily attained. Even when the wires have been placed into one bone there is a tendency for the bone ends to move apart as they are inserted into the other bone. The space between them must therefore be filled before the wires can be removed. If efficient fixation occurs, there will be only minor callus formation and subsequent union may either be slow or the result of fibrous tissue formation. It has been our practice instead to use a Harrison-Nicolle intramedullary peg, which makes easier the accurate apposition of the bone ends and is postoperatively more convenient for the patient. There are no projecting wires which have to be removed later and activity is permissible after only a short period of fixation. Relatively stable union is rapidly achieved even though, as with all forms of rigid internal fixation, complete bony union may not occur for several months. A number of special instruments have been devised to enable insertion of the peg but these are not essential.

As well as the usual surgical foundation set which may include (SHH) a Harrison needle-holder and dissecting forceps, the following may be added: a Mitchell's scaler, or trimmer for making the initial perforation of the bone; a bone nibbler; two

Harrison bone-hooks; four graded Nicolle reamers (a size 7 is usually used for terminal joints); a Harrison bone-holding forceps; and two straight Spencer Wells artery clips. A drill is also required, especially if cortical bone has encroached the cancellous zone and it is difficult to prepare the cavity through the cortical bone by reamer alone. However, a fine drill with cutting blade can be easily used in all cases to replace the reamers if this is preferred. Intramedullary pegs are made in a number of sizes and angles (**Figure 8.2**). A terminal joint usually requires a 25° peg. A similar fixation angle will be required if crossed K-wires are used.

8.3

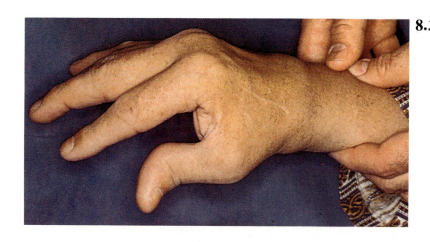

8.3

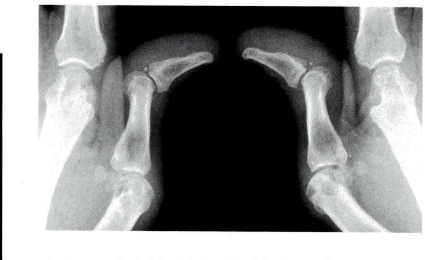

8.2

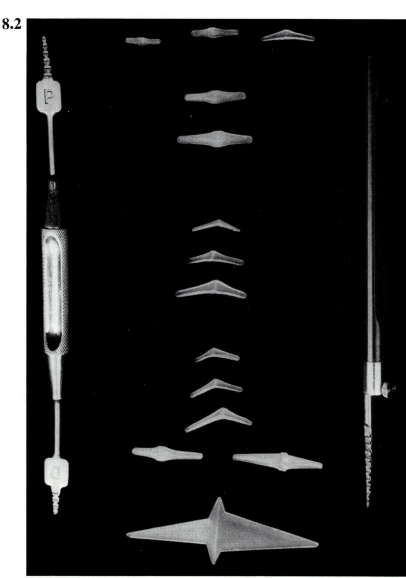

8.2 A range of Harrison-Nicolle polypropylene pegs in sizes (top to bottom) small, medium and large, in angles of 25°, 30°, 40°, and 50°. Below are straight pegs, sizes large and extra large above a wrist peg. On the left is a Nicolle reamer and on the right a Harrison reamer and handle.

Restoration of pinch by joint fixation following tendon rupture
As an alternative to tendon grafting, in cases in which the long flexor tendons to both thumb and index finger have been ruptured, fusion of the joints can effect a satisfactory pinch relationship.

8.3a Rheumatoid arthritis in a middle-aged patient who had ruptured the tendons of both the thumb and index finger in both hands. The index finger can be seen to be flexed at the metacarpophalangeal joint and hyperextended at the proximal interphalangeal joint. The thumb is flexed at the metacarpophalangeal joint and there is well-marked hyperextension of the terminal joint.

8.3b The extent of the hyperextension is clearly demonstrated in the X-ray of the terminal joint of the thumb; it has progressed to a dorsal subluxation. Passive flexion has been lost and therefore there was no hope of restoring an active range of movement by inserting a tendon graft.

8.3c A 25° angled peg has been inserted into the terminal joints of both thumb and the index finger and a 40° angled peg inserted into the proximal interphalangeal joint of the index finger. Adequate pinch has been restored. A similar procedure was performed on the opposite hand and function improved dramatically.

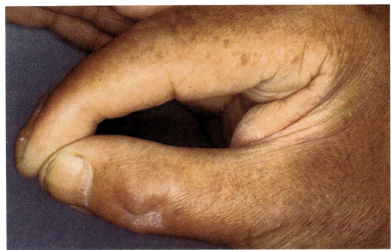

8.3c

The thumb metacarpophalangeal joint

This joint commonly requires arthrodesis. Flexion deformity is a common complaint and is usually followed by compensatory hyperextension deformity of the interphalangeal joint. One cause of the deformity lies in the disorganized and stretched extensor apparatus and joint ligaments. Soft-tissue reparative procedures do not usually improve the condition; if there is good carpometacarpal control, arthrodesis is the most effective treatment. Arthrodesis is also required in cases of painful joint destruction (**Figure 8.3**), particularly when this is associated with extensor or flexor tendon rupture (see Chapter 7). One of the earliest deformities in rheumatoid arthritis is adduction of the first metacarpal joint. This deformity is secondary to carpometacarpal joint disease and can also occur in osteoarthrosis. As the thumb becomes adducted, pinch between thumb and index finger alters from opposition to apposition, thus the finger meets the side of the thumb rather than the pad in opposition. This side-to-side pinch leads to increased strain on the side of the thumb, whose metacarpophalangeal joint may also be subject to joint disease, so producing weakening, stretch and ultimately rupture of the ulnar collateral ligament of the first metacarpophalangeal joint. This, in turn, produces radial instability and deviation (**Figure 8.4**).

8.4

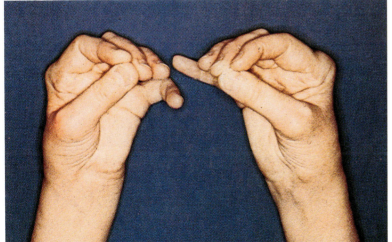

The carpometacarpal joint

This joint is the axial joint for thumb activity and as such it is particularly vulnerable to rheumatoid involvement among the arthropathies. It is also especially vulnerable to osteoarthrosis, either as a primary condition or secondary to an arthropathy, or to trauma as, for example, following a Bennett's fracture. The problem is worsened in rheumatoid disease by collapse of the ligamentous control and often of the trapezium itself so that the metacarpal base falls from its trapezial support and the metacarpal moves into adduction deformity; this problem may be worsened by secondary shortening of the structures in the thumb web space.

Since the basic synovial effects are not dramatic a simple synovectomy is rarely performed, and surgical support tends to be limited to states of frank joint destruction and thumb disability.

Treatment by mobility is acceptable if an effective web space distance can be achieved and the thumb is maintained thus in full activity. It is also needed if the distal joints have had to be fixed previously for any reason. There are various recommendable forms of treatment. If the trapezium itself gives good support to the thumb and the problem is essentially one of damaged surfaces (as, for example, after a Bennett's fracture in a younger person), it is often worth trying a thin silicone rubber or similar insert between the metacarpal and the trapezium. This should be sutured in while repairing the capsule, otherwise it will be unstable and move.

With the enthusiasm for silicone rubber replacements the trapezium itself is often so replaced. Unfortunately, the trapezium is firmly held into the carpus by strong ligaments, particularly on its deep aspect (hence the difficulty in removing the bone). Thus, the implant is basically unstable. Various complicated techniques have been developed to improve the situation but in our experience these seem hardly justified when the final result is a minimal improvement on a simple trapeziectomy – an operation which gives excellent long-term results. After trapeziectomy the thumb drops slightly, and the remainder of the space vacated by bone fills with fibrous tissue, so giving, in effect, a fibrous arthroplasty.

The operation is not easy because there is the problem of removing a bone which is locked in its deepest part to the remaining carpus by a process and a strong ligament. Consequently, separation is rather difficult: the bone surfaces will almost certainly exhibit considerable roughness and joint space will be lost due to osteoarthrosis.

Removal of the bone in one piece, as described, is the best method but in cases where this appears unduly difficult it is advisable to remove it by gradual nibbling with bone nibblers. Using the latter method it is important that all the trapezium, particularly its deep process, is removed.

Trapeziometacarpal arthrodesis is recommended in some cases, especially where the osteoarthrosis is limited to that joint, as for example, following a Bennett's fracture. Excision, however, is more suitable when there is more general involvement. The operative procedure for arthrodesis is similar to the early stages of excision (up to stage 9) – see pages 167 to 169.

The epiphysis at the base of the thumb can be affected in cases of seronegative juvenile polyarthritis (Still's disease). This was the only apparent manifestation in the hand of the patient

8.5a

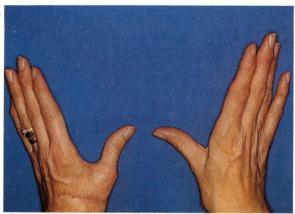

8.5b

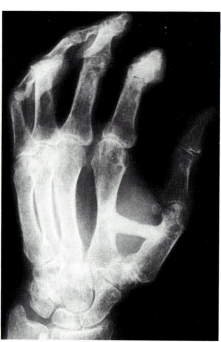

8.5a A patient with seronegative juvenile arthritis in childhood which led to progressive adduction deformity due to involvement of the thumb metacarpal epiphysis. The right hand still shows the deformity but the left has been treated by an intermetacarpal bone graft.

8.5b The graft is well consolidated and the carpometacarpal joint has also fused.

shown in **Figures 8.5a** and **8.5b**. She developed a progressive adduction deformity of the thumb 25 years after onset. If a bone graft is inserted between the first and second metacarpals, as shown in **Figures 8.5a** and **8.5b**, and similarly in degenerative arthritis, it will correct any adduction deformity and immobilize the carpometacarpal joint. Pain will be relieved and the subsequent loss of movement will not seriously incapacitate the patient. When the joint space is narrowed, a small sheet of silastic may be inserted between the joint surfaces in order to prevent fusion occurring. This is known as the 'bypass operation' (SHH).

A similar operation can be performed in rheumatoid cases: the adduction deformity has been corrected after the graft has been tapped into place.

As an alternative to a bone graft, two straight polypropylene pegs (large and extra large respectively), can be inserted into holes in the two metacarpals so that they lie parallel. This method is satisfactory for the correction of adduction deformity in rheumatic patients, but does not provide the perfect immobilization of a bone graft. Slight movement at the carpometacarpal joint may give rise to pain in cases of degenerative arthritis.

If the first metacarpophalangeal joint is deformed, and the joint eroded, it should be stabilized with a straight peg at the same operation especially if there is effective control and movement of the interphalangeal joint.

The fingers

The metacarpophalangeal joint in the finger is the axial joint and hence most likely to be involved in and eventually distorted and destroyed by rheumatoid and other arthropathies. As digital control depends upon an effectively controlled metacarpophalangeal joint, its disorganization must have secondary effects upon the interphalangeal joints. They may themselves also show destructive changes. Thus interphalangeal joint disorganization can come directly from joint or periarticular

change of itself, from metacarpophalangeal disorganization, or from both. The problem of analysing the mechanism of, and the correct treatment for what appears to be interphalangeal joint disorganization can thus be considerable, requiring much clinical skill and experience. In general however, the conditions found can be grouped into either joint collapse or abnormal control.

The distal interphalangeal joints
The terminal joints of the fingers are most commonly affected in osteoarthrosis (degenerative arthritis) and psoriatic arthropathy. The latter tends to be a destructive disease of joints, frequently leading to severe instability which can be most incapacitating; it may, however, go the other way and produce joint fixation, leaving the finger joints in abnormal and unacceptable positions.

The techniques of terminal interphalangeal joint arthrodesis have already been described for the thumb and this is equally applicable to the finger.

The proximal interphalangeal joints
These joints can also become deformed and unstable or abnormally fixed. In such cases the treatment is likely to be arthrodesis in an optimal position. When finger joint prostheses first became available it was often recommended that they were ideal for interphalangeal replacement. Now even the most ardent supporters of prostheses for the metacarpophalangeal joints have generally accepted that they are not suitable for the interphalangeal joint and that arthrodesis is to be preferred.

Many deformities of the proximal interphalangeal joints are the result of widely differing pathology, often outside the joint; they can be flexion, extension, or lateral deformities.

Flexion deformity. The term Boutonnière is often used loosely to describe any flexion deformity of the proximal interphalangeal joint. It should be discarded except for the condition it specifically describes, which is a tear of the extensor tendon from its insertion to the base of the middle phalanx, in which the head of the proximal phalanx presents in the gap. As a result of the retraction of the central slip of the extensor tendon, the intrinsic tendons, which are attached to the central tendon, are retracted proximally. There is relative shortening of the intrinsics, and the terminal joint becomes hyperextended.

Flexion deformity of the proximal interphalangeal joint in the rheumatoid hand is frequently not associated with a hyperextension deformity of the terminal joint. This is presumptive evidence that the central tendon is intact but stretched, and rupture is rarely the cause of the deformity. Hyperextension of the terminal joint in these cases can occur from a passive extension force, as happens in the 'Z' deformity of the thumb.

There is a much higher incidence of flexion deformity in

juveniles (particularly seronegative juvenile polyarthritis), whereas swan's-neck deformity is much more common in adults. When present in adults with rheumatoid disease, it is a progressive deformity of the joint itself; in children it is often due to flexor tendon disease. In seronegative juvenile poly- arthritis, epiphyseal involvement is common, and is associated with collapse of the articular surface. This can progress to a flexion deformity of the proximal interphalangeal joint.

Flexion deformity, when associated with proliferative synovitis, is an indication for a synovectomy, although the operation itself will not improve the flexion deformity but will reduce its likely progress towards the condition shown in **Figure 8.6**.

Attempts to repair the extensor tendon in these cases is not usually effective, although a 'tuck' in the central slip over the proximal phalanx may delay the progress to deformity. The finger should be maintained in interphalangeal extension for three weeks after synovectomy or repair if there is lengthening of the central slip.

8.6

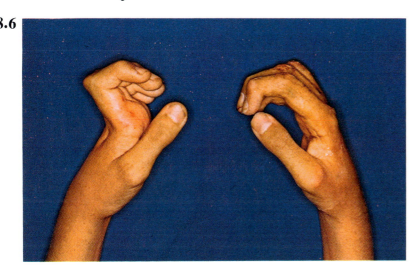

Swan's-neck or hyperextension deformity can be aetiologically classified thus:
1 volar plate
2 intra-articular
3 extra-articular
    (a) subluxation of the metacarpophalangeal joint in the anteroposterior plane.
    (b) dislocation of the extensor tendon.
Swan's-neck deformity can occur as a result of loss of the free gliding of the volar plate, in much the same way as it occurs following loss of the action of the check ligament, due to trauma (Harrison 1960).

The synovial proliferation fills the joint and lines the volar plate. It is extruded out of the joint into the check ligament, and the mechanism which controls extension of the joint loses the ability to recoil after extension; as a result, extension strain allows progressive extension deformity.

Intra-articular progressive joint destruction is associated with partial detachment of the ligaments, which control the stability of the proximal interphalangeal joints, and in such cases extension strain permits hyperextension of the joint and limits the recoil. These cases are not infrequently seen in juvenile rheumatoid arthritis.

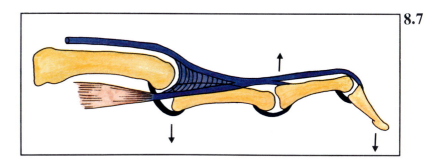

8.7

When the flexion of the deformity is established and exceeds 45°, the treatment of choice is stabilization of the joint, using an angled intramedullary peg or other form of fixation.

This type of deformity is also seen in the 'main en griffe' deformity, where both ulnar and median nerves have been divided. It can be seen in scleroderma and in syringo-myelia. In all these cases, the cause lies mainly in the flexor tendon, rather than the joint.

Acute flexion of a proximal interphalangeal joint can occur; if this affects a single joint it is more characteristic of Still's disease than of adult rheumatoid arthritis. It does, however, sometimes follow flexor tenosynovitis, i.e. a secondary fixed trigger finger (see Chapter 5). Such cases are best treated by stabilization.

In the rheumatoid hand, flexion deformity of up to 45° is acceptable but any further flexion should be treated by stabilization.

Extra-articular causes are probably the most common in swan's-neck deformity in adults and often secondary to sub- luxation of the metacarpophalangeal joints (**Figure 8.7**).

Normally, extension strain on the flat hand is taken at the metacarpophalangeal joints, but if these are subluxated then the extension strain is taken at the proximal interphalangeal joint. *Extra-articular swan's-neck deformity* has three phases:
1 actively reducible subluxation
2 passively reducible subluxation
3 irreducible subluxation.
Actively reducible subluxation does not require treatment other than to overcome aggravating factors. Passively reducible subluxation can be controlled, at least temporarily, by dividing one intrinsic tendon proximally, at the level of the base of the proximal phalanx, dissecting it distally, then re-routing it through the volar plate, and ultimately suturing to itself (**Figure**

8.8

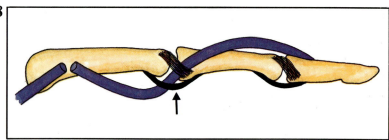

8.8). Littler originally used an intrinsic release, by dividing the junction fibres between the central tendon and the intrinsic, i.e. the wing tendon of the expansion, leaving the transverse fibres of the interosseous insertion intact, but the correction is often only temporary.

Irreducible swan's-neck deformity is best corrected by arthrodesis of the proximal interphalangeal joint at 45° of flexion. In those cases in which the metacarpophalangeal joints are subluxated, it is desirable to correct that deformity by arthroplasty at the same time, or in two stages.

8.9

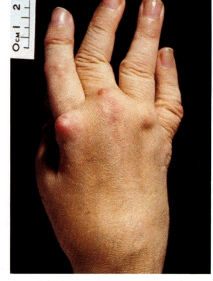

8.9 *Lateral instability* is more often seen in juvenile rheumatoid arthritis, although lateral deformity is not uncommon in adults and can also occur in psoriatic arthropathy. The deformity is due to joint destruction, and may be painful; furthermore it can alter the mechanism of pinch and will necessitate functional correction.

The treatment for both instability and deformity is arthrodesis.

The metacarpophalangeal joints

These are, as already stressed, the prime joints of the fingers and must be protected from damage as early as is reasonably possible, by such means as synovectomy. It is also important to attempt to maintain effective power in the main supporting muscles, the interossei. This will in turn influence the extensor expansion and limit stretching, particularly in its weakest part between the radial sided interosseous muscle and the extensor tendon (a primary cause of ulnar drift). The radial sided interosseous becomes at mechanical disadvantage and weak-

ness. If however its strength can be maintained, so also may the radial side of the extensor expansion. The so-called 'crab-walk' (KMB) can be very valuable in maintaining the necessary joint support (**Figure 8.10**). Any attempts at soft tissue realignment should be preceded and followed by radial deviating exercises of the fingers.

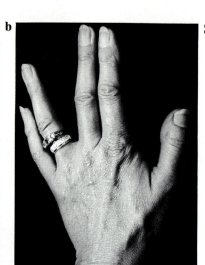

8.10 **'Crab-walk' radial deviating exercise.** The hand is laid on a surface with fingers straight or bent, whichever is easier and the fingers successively carried into radial deviation with maximal effort. The process is repeated – the hand thus crab-walking across the surface.

Metacarpophalangeal joint realignment can often be valuable, particularly if the above exercise support is given to strengthen both the muscles and the other periarticular tissues.

There are three aspects of realignment to be considered:
1 The analysis of function; the change from the normal to the abnormal.
2 The chain-reaction to deformity; one deformity will lead to another unless the progress is interrupted.
3 The mode of repair; at what stage and by what means can the insidious loss of function be interrupted?

The surgical indications are:
1 To preserve function.
2 To recognize and interrupt the chain-reaction.
3 To restore function.

The functional relationship of the thumb to the fingers is the most important requirement in the hand. Power grip, particularly in rheumatoid patients, may be relatively unimportant as they may not be called upon to do heavy work, and so require only a limited capacity to hold and to lift. The primary objectives therefore are to restore and maintain the ability to pinch and perform precise movements between the thumb and fingers, particularly the index and middle. The index finger also requires the support of the middle finger in strong lateral pinch, to prevent it giving way under the pressure of the apposing thumb. Initially the middle finger is commonly the first digit to show evidence of ulnar drift and, when established, its lack of support for the index finger is sufficiently important to warrant surgical interference.

The little finger is the next common digit to drift, often due to the presence of a bursa or, to be more accurate, synovial bulk within the joint which erodes into the bone on the head of the fifth metacarpal, causing partial detachment of the collateral ligament and, in particular, stretching of the radial side of the expansion and inducing dislocation of the extensor tendon ulnarwards. This feature occurs in all fingers but appears more dramatically in the little finger. Also, at the point of insertion of the extensor, through the dorsal plate to the base of the phalanx, erosions may occur which may lead to detachment of the plate, thus producing, with the stretched collateral ligaments, anterior subluxation of the phalanx on the metacarpal head (**Figure 8.11**).

The mode of repair will depend upon the grade of deformity (see page 26).

The reconstruction of grades 1 and 2, i.e. early ulnar drift, is

.11

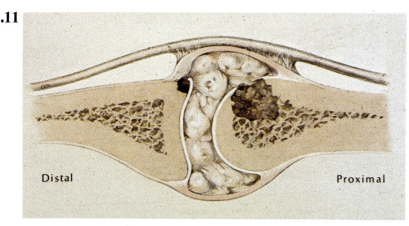

8.11 On the dorsum of the head of the metacarpal some erosive change can be seen. On the radial side of the head an erosion or geode would imply, since it would be close to the attachment of the collateral ligament, detachment or impending detachment of the ligament thus permitting volar subluxation.

best done by some form of realignment, the principles being:
1 Centralization of the extensor tendon.
2 Reconstruction of a functioning extensor mechanism.
3 Correction of the ulnar drift by intrinsic transfer.
4 Reinforcement of the radial collateral ligament.
Two methods will be described.

The first offers (SHH) greater mechanical stability and is to

be recommended where effective preoperative and postoperative physiotherapeutic control cannot be guaranteed.

The second, a rather simpler method, can be valuable (KMB) but it is essential that before the operation the patient must have effective training of the radial sided interossei (**Figure 8.10**). The reasons why simple intrinsic transfers fail in many hands are:
1 Failure to build up the strength of those muscles which will have become ineffective as the periarticular disruption has progressed.
2 Failure to involve and support the radial collateral ligaments.
3 Incorrect placement of the transferred tendon.

With these provisos the simpler operation can give excellent results with the minimum of reorganization in a well-motivated patient. It is in fact a simple extension of a metacarpophalangeal synovectomy.

In grade 3 deformity there may be soft tissue shortening and it may not be possible to correct the subluxation without shortening the bone – as in an excision arthroplasty – by removal of the metacarpal head. There is often adaptive shortening on the flexor aspect, and it is necessary to release the flexor tendon from the digital theca and divide the shortened ulnar intrinsic. Sometimes it is possible by serial plasters and other physiotherapeutic stretching techniques to pull out the muscular shortening but this must be done with care and any leverage of the fingers to further stress the already stretched metacarpophalangeal joint tissues should be carefully avoided.

In group 3 cases, where the subluxation has proved difficult to correct, despite extensive soft tissue release, and in group 4 cases, where the subluxation causes limited extension, interposition arthroplasty becomes necessary, so that the correction can be maintained. It is particularly important to observe this criterion of treatment because if ulnar drift is corrected, but not subluxation, then the proximal interphalangeal joints will be subject to repeated extension strain, which will ultimately leads to swan's-neck deformities and a disability far greater than an ulnar drift (**Figure 8.12**).

A number of prostheses have been designed for the metacarpophalangeal joints – the Flatt metal articulated prosthesis; the Swanson flexible silastic prosthesis; the Niebauer Dacron-incorporated prosthesis; the Calnan–Nicolle polypropylene prosthesis, and many more. These are all designed to correct the subluxation, maintain the corrected alignment of the fingers and allow movement in flexion and extension. We have

8.12

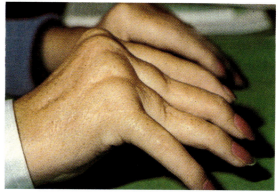

usually used the Swanson prosthesis; the method of its insertion will be described but that of most other types is very similar.

Most descriptions of the insertion of metacarpophalangeal joint prostheses tend to neglect the supportive soft tissues. There is a tendency to cut and leave shortened interossei. It has long been the practice of both surgical authors to combine insertion of a prosthesis with a soft-tissue manoeuvre to give maximal dynamic support to the new joint.

In our experience, the results with this extra support have been far superior to a simple joint replacement. It is interesting to note that dissatisfaction with the simple type of operation has caused many surgeons to use soft tissue supportive surgery.

Although in theory the various hinge prostheses would appear to give all that is needed for joint replacement, they all fall far short of the functional quality achieved from, say, a good hip prosthesis. In the latter case there is an efficient ball and socket with excellent all round muscle activity and control. In the finger, control is largely through the tendons, with the muscles some distance away. Hence in the simple hinge of interphalangeal joints where theoretically a replacement hinge should be satisfactory, the results have generally been found to be unsatisfactory and arthrodesis is now generally preferred in the majority of cases. Even where there are no soft tissue problems the joints tends to stiffen, as also happens in the metacarpophalangeal joints; reports of prosthesis fracture are becoming common.

As an alternative to the use of permanent interposition materials to maintain the arthroplasty and to avoid foreign materials being maintained permanently in the joint area it has become our practice to maintain the correction of subluxation and ulnar drift by the use of straight pegs. These are inserted as a temporary measure for 10 days or so, and then removed (SHH). The rationale behind this technique is that although prostheses have been carefully designed to act as hinges, they very soon become surrounded by heavy scar tissue as shown in the post mortem specimen of a Swanson prosthesis about one year after insertion (**Figure 8.13**).

The prosthesis no longer serves its original purpose but merely forms the core of a fibrous arthroplasty. If therefore the bones are maintained stable in good position until a fibrous union forms, the foreign body can be removed. The results have been as good as with a retained prosthetic joint and the cost is merely that of a simple polypropylene peg – a fraction of the cost of most joint prostheses.

8.13

8.13 A Swanson prosthesis is shown firmly embedded in fibrous tissue in a post-mortem specimen. It forms no more than a silastic core to a fibrous arthroplasty, a frequent result of a finger prosthesis. As can be seen, the design of the prosthesis (below) carefully developed to allow flexion, has been made ineffective by fibrosis.

Arthrodesis of the wrist

A degree of fixation or complete arthrodesis of the wrist can be a most valuable form of treatment, not only in rheumatoid and similar arthropathies where there may be joint collapse, but also in painful osteoarthrosis. Although a degree of flexion is useful in a few activities (e.g. toiletry) by far the greater part of wrist movement is to ulnar deviation with the forearm held in the mid prone position (e.g. use of a light hammer, power grip, etc.). This activity is usually in the same plane as elbow movement and thus wrist movement can be obliterated (as it is normally for use of a heavier hammer) so long as the elbow moves satisfactorily and there is effective pronation and supination.

Collapse of the wrist complex is common in rheumatoid disease but so also is the tendency for the wrist to fix in unacceptable positions. Fixed radial deviation, probably initiated as a protective measure due to involvement of the distal radio ulnar joint, has been said to be responsible for ulnar drift of the fingers but the conditions are likely to be co-existent rather than directly linked. In seronegative juvenile polyarthritis or Still's disease an early sign of the condition can be a fixed flexed wrist. If this is not corrected early (by splinting etc.) then the deformity will become permanent.

The concept of synovectomy of the wrist followed by a period of immobilization has been described in Chapter 6 and this certainly helps a considerable proportion of patients with wrist disorganization. Such a procedure is, however, unlikely to help if there is a considerable amount of volar collapse. If there is severe wrist and mid carpal destruction, arthrodesis is the treatment of choice. However, in a proportion of the less severe cases a removal of the proximal carpal row at the same time as a synovectomy of the remaining joints followed by a period of immobilisation in a good position will often give excellent results. The patient then has a small amount of residual movement in an acceptable position so long as the hand has been set up in a good position at the operation.

There is a wide variety of methods of wrist arthrodesis, which must lead to fixation of the radius either directly or through carpal remnants to the index and middle fingers – the stable axis of the hand. The ulna must not be included and wherever possible, pronation and supination must be maintained.

Whatever the technique, the joint surface must be cut back to cancellous bone and then fixed until bony union has occurred. This can be achieved effectively by external (plaster) fixation supported, if necessary, by a bone graft. A rib graft is useful and can give the needed curve of the wrist in gentle flexion or an ileal graft can give whichever curve is required.

(A degree of dorsiflexion is ideal for function but if both wrists are to be fixed one must be in a degree of flexion or personal toiletry becomes impossible.) If the distal end of the ulna is to be removed at the same time, as, for example, where there is pronation/supination blocking, small pieces can be used as packing.

Internal fixation techniques such as A.O. and similar plates can be useful in osteoarthrosis but it must be remembered that in rheumatoid disease the bones are likely to have a consistency little firmer than butter and even cancellous screws cut out. In these cases a Steinman pin or Rush nail can be passed through the index or middle finger metacarpal head, whichever is better

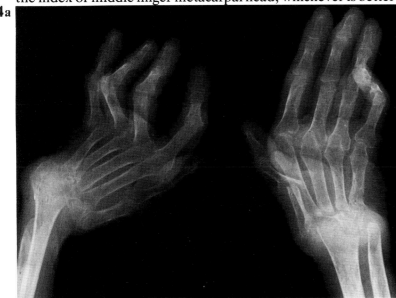

14a

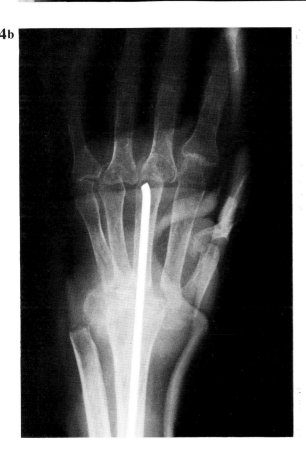

.14b

for position, through into the radius. The end of the pin or nail (the hook should be cut off the Rush nail) should be pushed below the joint surface of the metacarpal head. A Rush nail is softer and can be bent a little at the wrist to give a curve as required but this must not be attempted if the bone is too soft (**Figure 8.14**).

There is some argument as to whether the index or middle finger metacarpal should be used for the pin or nail. Those who favour the index finger tend to support this on the grounds that the wrist should not show radial deviation, as this is said to aggravate ulnar drift of the fingers. This argument is probably not entirely valid since the difference in angulation is slight. If the patient has an effective power grip potential there is something to be said for a degree of ulnar deviation in fixation which can be achieved through the index metacarpal. From a practical point of view, in most cases of rheumatoid disease at least, the choice depends more on the state of the bones than on other considerations. In osteoarthrosis, the hand may show much greater potential to function with a fixed wrist and therefore the accurate positioning with slight ulnar deviation and extension is more important (so long as one wrist is available into flexion for toiletry).

An excellent alternative method of internal fixation can be achieved by using a Harrison polypropylene peg which by reversing can give either a dorsal or volar curve at the wrist of 25°, and the technique will be described in a patient who had juvenile rheumatoid disease, disorganized wrists with flexion deformity and ruptured extensor digital tendons.

Removal of the trapezium

Synovitis leading to collapse of the capsule and/or the joint surfaces is often the precursor of considerable thumb deformity and functional loss. Osteoarthritic changes either from the inflammatory diseases or from osteoarthrosis may reduce hand function due to thumb base pain. The thumb metacarpal may become subluxated on the trapezium which tends to carry the thumb in to the hand and reduce web distance. Alternatively a similar effect commonly occurs due to the patient protecting the thumb against the pain. The end result of both is secondary shortening of the thumb web space structures.

As the basic synovial effects are not dramatic a simple synovectomy is rarely carried out and so surgical support tends to be limited to states of frank joint destruction and thumb disability.

The treatment for such a condition can be a trapeziectomy. The thumb drops slightly and the remainder of the space vacated by the bone fills with fibrous tissue, so giving a fibrous pad.

More recently, with the enthusiasm for prosthetics, the bone once removed has been replaced by one of silastic or other

— Continued on page 166

8.14a and 8.14b This patient had complete collapse of the wrist and all extensor tendons were ruptured, only the two extensor carpi radialis tendons remaining intact. The ulna projected as a large knob dorsally. The joint was excised, a Rush nail passed through the middle metacarpal and the ulnar head used as bone graft chips. The extensor carpi radialis longus was used as motor to the thumb and the brevis to the fingers, giving good function.

Arthrodesis of the thumb interphalangeal joint

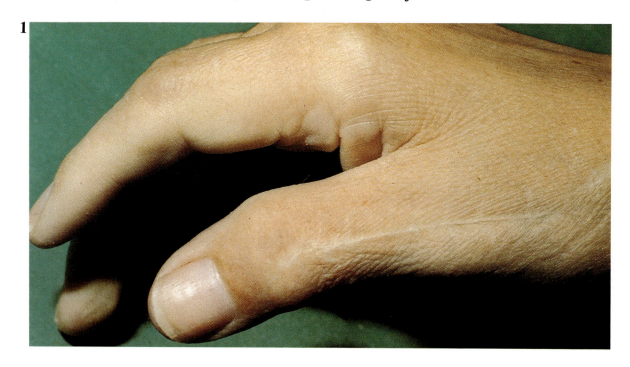

1 The joint is deviated, painful and grossly unstable, thus requiring correction and stabilization. The scar along the dorsum of the thumb is the site of a previous operation for the insertion of a straight peg into the first metacarpophalangeal joint, for a flexion deformity from joint destruction due to rheumatoid arthritis.

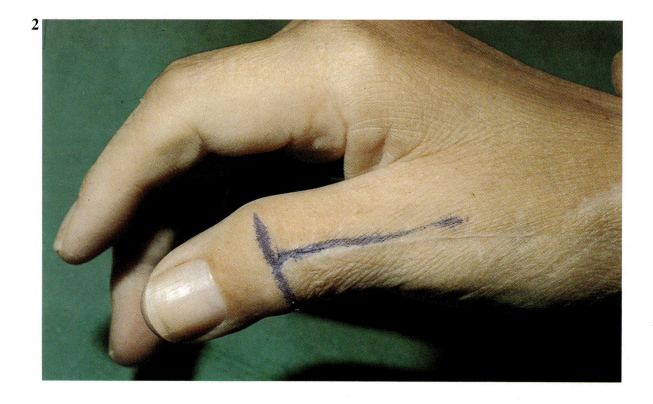

2 The T-shaped incision is made possible by the excellent vascular anastomosis around the nail bed, and has greatly facilitated the problems of arthrodesis of the terminal joint, both in the thumb and fingers. The stages of this operation are the same in a terminal finger joint.

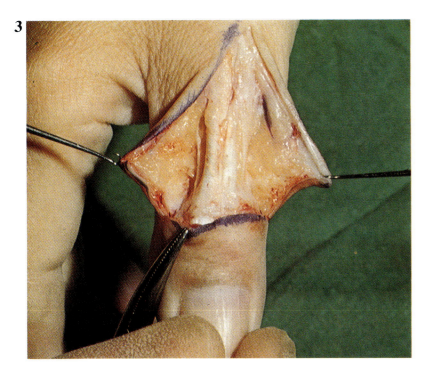

3 A tourniquet is applied. After elevation of skin flaps, the extensor tendon is exposed and the distal skin edge slightly undermined. This must not be too extensive or the nail bed may be damaged.

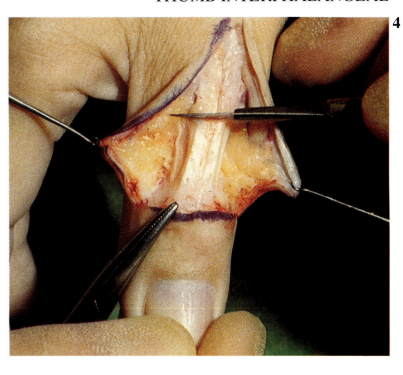

4 The extensor tendon is divided proximal to the joint and should be retained for suturing postoperatively.

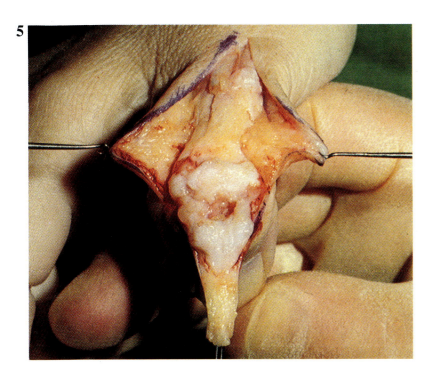

5 A stay stitch is inserted into the distal cut tendon, and after dissecting this distally, it will act as a retractor. Gross destructive changes can be seen in the joint.

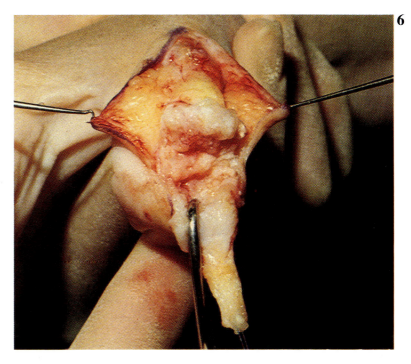

6 The sharp bone-hook is inserted into the articular surface of the terminal phalanx for retraction, to facilitate the dissection of the soft tissue attachments.

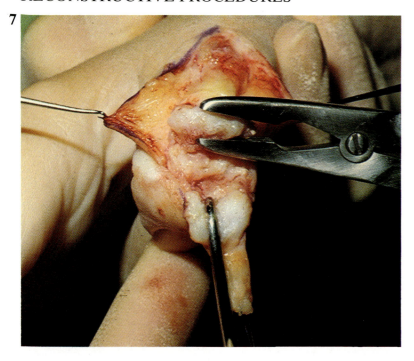

7 The remnants of articular cartilage are removed from both joint surfaces with a bone nibbler, so that the bone ends will fit accurately together at an angle of 25°.

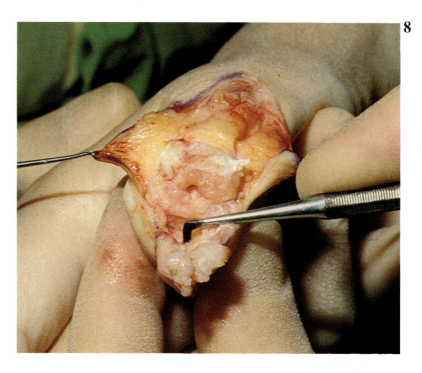

8 If using pegs the bone ends are initially perforated with the sharp end of the Mitchell's scaler or trimmer.

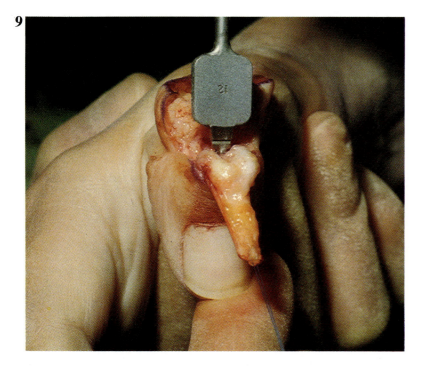

9 The distal end of a number 7 Nicholle reamer is inserted into the distal phalanx, and a suitable cavity reamed out to accommodate the stem of the peg. Alternatively this can be carried out with a fine cutting or reciprocating drill (**Figure 4**, page 177).

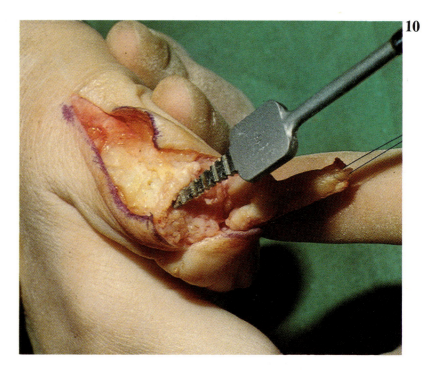

10 A similar procedure is performed on the proximal phalanx, using the proximal end of the reamer. The reamer should be thrust in and out of the cavity, and any angulation avoided, otherwise the end of the reamer can break off in the cavity. If this happens, a drill hole is made proximally in the dorsal aspect of the bone, and the broken reamer is pushed out from proximal to distal.

11

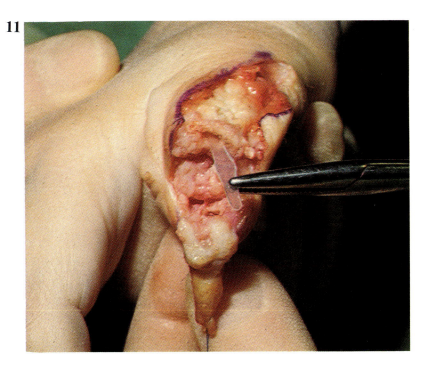

11 A 25° angled peg is first inserted into the proximal phalanx up to the shoulder of the central section of the peg.

12

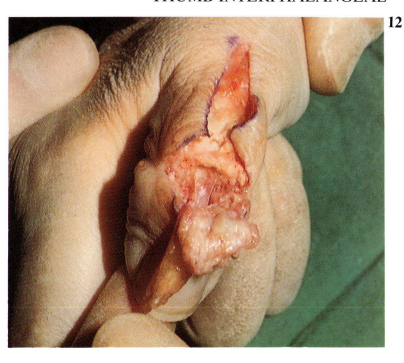

12 The peg is now in place proximally, and the distal end will enter the cavity in the terminal phalanx without difficulty, provided that adequate distraction of the base of the terminal phalanx can be provided by the sharp hook and stay suture, and that the base of the phalanx has been adequately cleared of its soft tissue attachments.

13

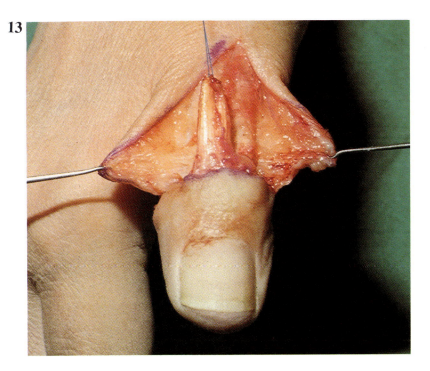

13 After compacting the bone junction (whether using peg or K-wires), the extensor tendon is repaired by suture, thus providing good cover and stability.

14

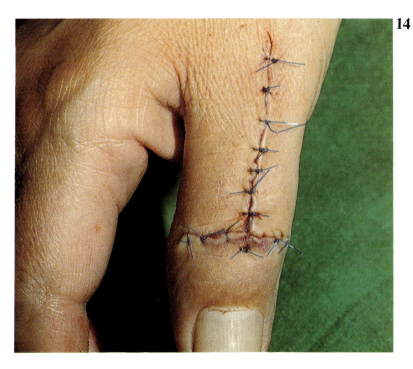

14 The wound is closed.

15

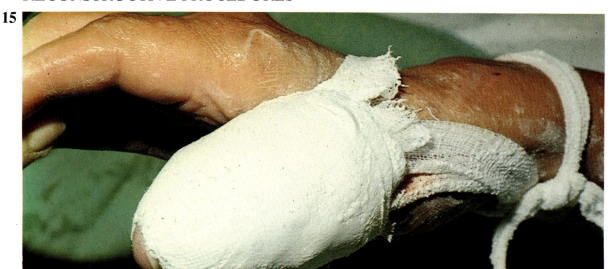

15 A dressing, reinforced with a plaster of Paris or similar splint is required for four to six weeks. The terminal pulp should be visible for inspection.

16

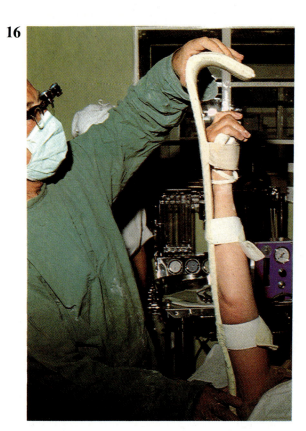

17

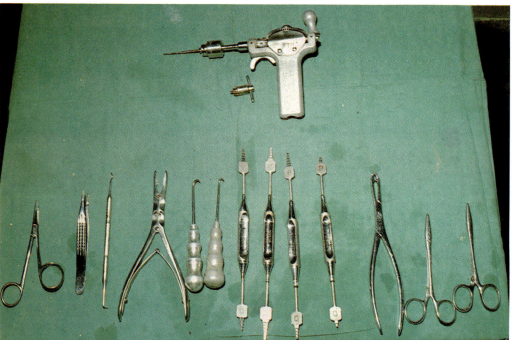

16 The tourniquet should be released before wound closure, and haemostasis established. There should be no unnecessary delay in elevating the arm, and this should be established in the operating theatre and maintained until the postoperative oedema has subsided in three to four days' time, or whenever the circumstances demand. This splint was designed and made in the hospital, and consists of 10 cm Cramer wire splinting, covered with adhesive felt. The limb is attached to the splint with Velcro bands. The top of the splint is angled and a bandage or cord suspends the splint to a blood stand. Alternatively a simple roller towel similarly suspended may be used with the arm pinned in as for all hand surgery.

17 Special instruments which are useful for carrying out an arthrodesis using Harrison–Nicolle pegs.

— *Continued from page 161*

material. Theoretically the idea is good for it gives the thumb a base on which it can move. In practice, however, the sheer forces and the relatively small fibrous response around the plastic has led to the prosthesis becoming unstable. A variety of procedures, sometimes fairly complicated, have been described to control the mobility of the prosthesis. The end results have been far better than the prosthesis alone but they appear to offer little improvement over a simple trapeziectomy. This latter is an excellent operation which has stood the test of time. There have been reports that although there is loss of pain, which also gives the patient a painless grip, there is also a loss of grip power. However, it is important, when considering such matters, to remember that whereas pinch grip gives considerable leverage effect at the thumb, the power grip uses the thumb mass; reported measurements of strength tend not to differen-

Excision of the trapezium

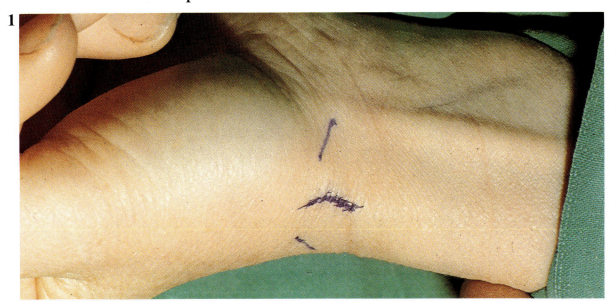

1 A satisfactory incision is made by following the crease lines at the base of the thumb. Relocation markers have been applied.

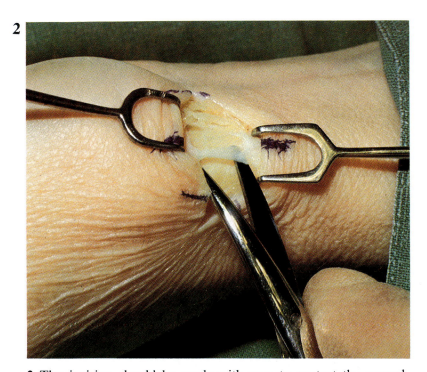

2 The incision should be made with care to protect the several underlying cutaneous nerve branches. These can be isolated by blunt dissection as shown.

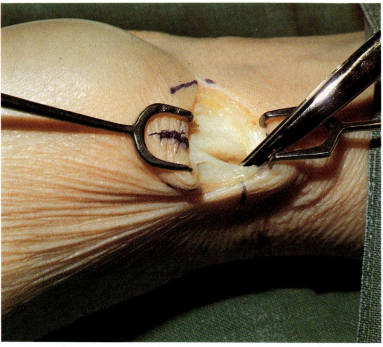

3 The nerves can be pushed outside by the double hook retractors. The blunt dissection can now progress into the anatomical snuffbox.

tiate effectively.

The operation is not easy in that there is the problem of removing a bone locked in its deepest part to the remaining carpus by a process and a strong ligament. This makes separation rather difficult especially as the bone surfaces will almost certainly exhibit considerable roughness and there will be loss of joint space due to osteoarthrosis.

It is always satisfying to remove the bone in one piece as is described, but where this appears unduly difficult it is advisable to remove it by gradual nibbling with bone nibblers, taking care that all the trapezium, and most particularly its deep process, is removed.

Sometimes trapeziometacarpal arthrodesis is recommended. This is a good operation if the osteoarthrosis is limited to that joint, as possibly after a Bennett's fracture, but excision is better for more general involvement. The operative procedure for arthrodesis is similar to that for excision in its early stages – i.e. up to **Figure 9**, page 169.

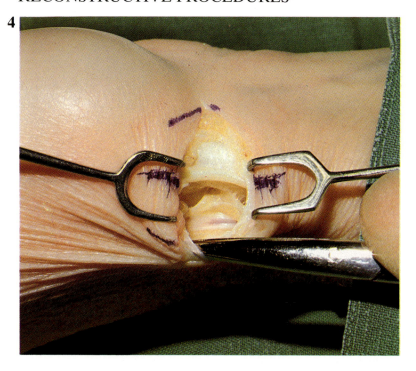

4 The tissues should be freed to the base of the metacarpal.

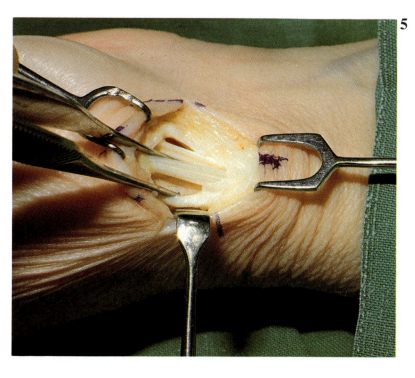

5 The abductor pollicis longus and extensor pollicis brevis tendons are identified.

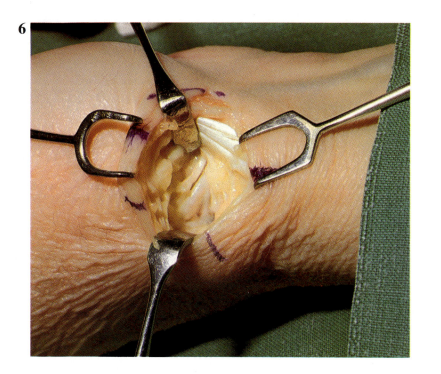

6 The radial artery must be identified in the base of the anatomical snuffbox.

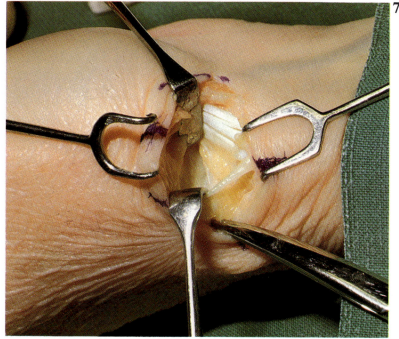

7 This can then be retracted, as can the tendons to allow access to the trapezium.

8

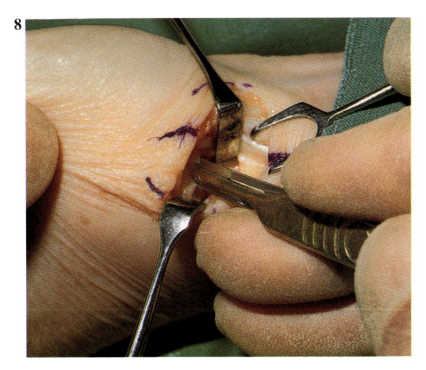

9

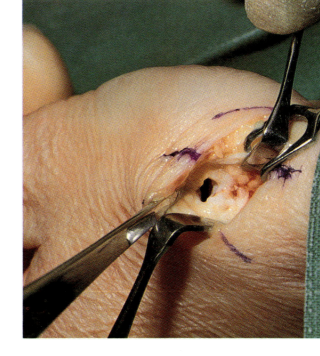

8 The carpometacarpal joint must now be identified.

9 If the hand is carried into full ulnar deviation this can be opened with ease and the trapezium is delivered more effectively to the operative field due to the rotation of the scaphoid below in this manoeuvre.

N.B. If a metacarpotrapezial arthrodesis is being performed the joint surfaces are now removed, the bones drilled and a graft applied.

10

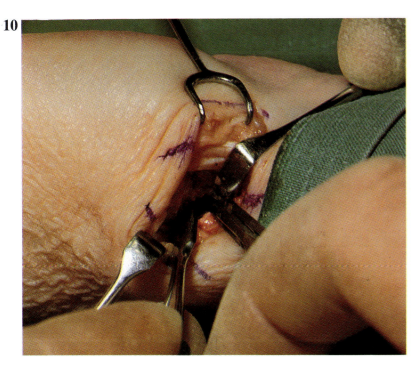

11

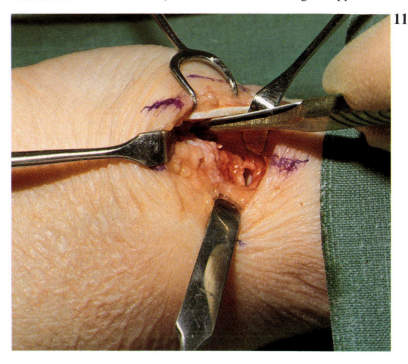

10 The ligaments of the carpometacarpal joint need to be divided in the depth of the joint. A McDonald elevator is being used to distract the joint surfaces and the assistant pulls out the thumb to give easier access.

11 The thenar muscles must now be separated from their origin on the volar aspect of the trapezium.

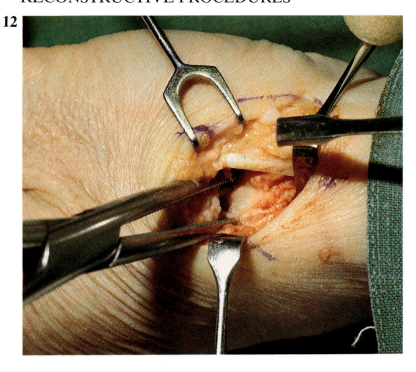

12 The dorsal and ventral surfaces of the bone are now free and can be grasped firmly.

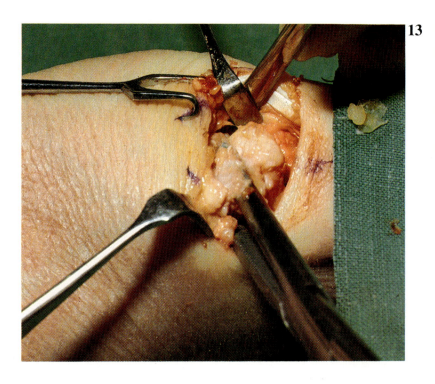

13 The ligaments on all sides and particularly in the depths must be divided, the bone being twisted in various directions as this is performed.

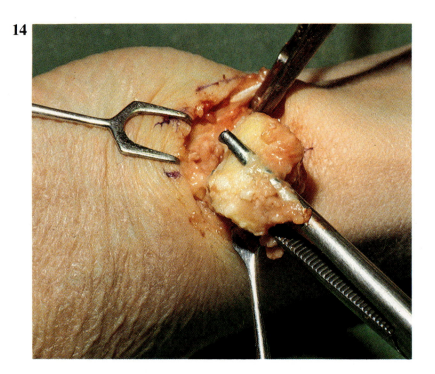

14 The bone is now free and is removed.

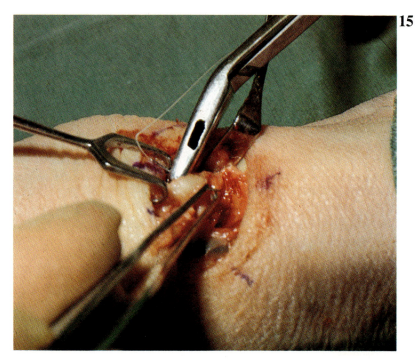

15 The thenar muscles are reattached and the capsular materials repaired.